Special Deliveries

Selecting the Gender of Your Baby
Before Conception

BOY OR GIRL?

By

Theresa Hebert

A simple, direct approach
to conceiving the child of your preference
supported by scientific research.

written: 1990
© copyright 1995
Third Edition 1998

DEDICATION

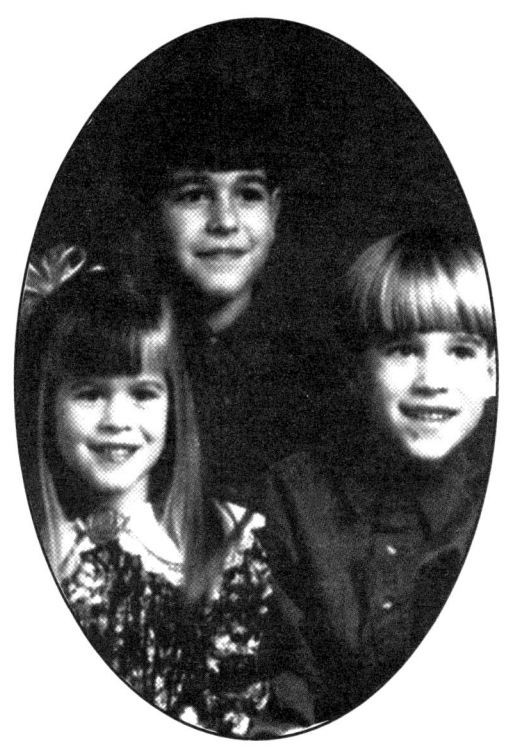

This book is lovingly dedicated to my three beautiful, very *"Special Deliveries,"* Alex Raymond, Brent Edward and Arielle Elena. You each have your own separate place in my heart. It's as if I grew a whole new heart when each of you were born.

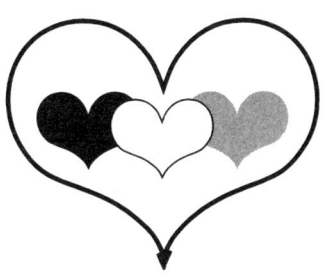

Special Deliveries
© copyright 1995
Revised 1998

Library of Congress catalogued, March 30, 1995

TXu 684 166

ISBN: 0-9648777-0-8

 Printed in the U.S.A.

Congratulations

"*Special Deliveries*" is very excited and happy for you. This book has already helped numerous couples achieve their desired results. Please read this book thoroughly, highlight all the pertinent information you have to adhere to, read it again, and then follow the procedures suggested. **Be patient until you feel confident.** If you aren't certain that you've grasped the entire method, don't be impatient. Go back and study what you've highlighted **until you are sure you are ready.**

If you conscientiously follow the instructions, you, too, will achieve your desired results. I wish you the best and eagerly look forward to hearing your individual success story!! Again, please take your time, be patient. The results are great ... **your precious bundle of joy.**

Wishing you much happiness,

Theresa   Hebert

CONSULT WITH THE AUTHOR

"*Special Deliveries*" is happy to announce, due to the tremendous volume of people wanting to communicate with the author, that we now offer phone consultations.

Personal Phone Consultation Fees:
FAX or Telephone (508) 880 - 7848
up to 20 minutes $20.00
Visa, Mastercard, Discover accepted

Return Mail Fee: $20.00

If you prefer to have your questions, relating to the book, answered by mail, we request that you enclose a self-addressed stamped envelope and a return mail fee of $20.00. Please make checks payable to "*Special Deliveries*".

"After I consult with people, I receive wonderful letters and comments like this":

I just wanted to thank you so very much for the book and all your help and knowledge. In speaking to you, you seem like such a wonderful person who's helping so many couples' dreams come true- you're an angel! This must be your calling in life (boy, I can't think of one that would make me feel so fulfilled). I plan on keeping in touch and will write you a note when I find out what gender my bundle of joy is! Take care and God bless you!

Sincerely,

Brenda L. Murphy

Perrysburg, Ohio

"Special Deliveries"
67 South Crane Ave.
Taunton, MA 02780

Dear Theresa:

It was great hearing you on the "Danny Bonaduce Show". It was also a pleasure to talk to you. I am so eager to read your book and I'm grateful that you thought enough of other people to publish it to help us!

Sincerely,
Terri J. Taylor
Detroit, Michigan

Dear Theresa:

I heard you talking about your book on "The Dave Ryan Radio Show" this morning, (in Minneapolis) and I must have a copy! I didn't get a chance to tell you on the phone that I do have a 5 year old daughter, and my husband and I have been trying for about two years now to have another baby. Being able to give myself a better chance of having a boy is an exciting thought. Thank you for being so nice on the phone. I think it's wonderful how you turned a difficult personal situation into a way to help others.

Sincerely,
Kera Lesure
St. Paul, Minnesota

Dear Theresa,

Thank you so much for talking to me today and for giving me confidence to be patient in trying for a little girl! My husband and I will keep trying and hopefully I can be included on your list of testimonials! You are such a positive person and I'm so glad I've had the opportunity to speak to you. Thank you again!

Fondly,
Kim Williams
Fairfield, Ohio

Since having been on national television, I have received some very positive affirming letters from professionals in the medical field, as well as the teaching field and religious life. They were all quite intrigued with my erudition. (Erudition being the learning acquired by researching and studying a particular subject matter.)

I've combined the theories of fertility doctors who have researched the subject of gender selection, some for well over 50 years with my own personal ideas, beliefs and findings. Some methods of timing support the *"Special Deliveries"* method of timing. However, *"Special Deliveries"* is proving that you can dispense with additional suggestions and simply concentrate your efforts on **timing** and still have the **safest, easiest,** most **natural** and best chance of conceiving the child of your preference.

Some doctors have suggested, for example, that women check their cervical mucus, yet most working women today are too busy to check their laundry or even prepare a meal for their families. They do not need **additional stress added to their lives!!** Being a busy working mother myself – I planned to keep it simple!! If, on the other hand, you are comfortable with this method by all means, what ever works for you.

NOTE: **You are the most fertile when the fluid in the cervical mucus is clear, slippery and stretchy with the consistency of an egg white. Following ovulation, the fluid dries up or thickens and feels more like rubber cement. Doctors caution that the cervical mucus method isn't surefire and should not be used alone. If a woman has irregular cycles or is not ovulating, it can be hard to read. Patients who don't ovulate may have what looks like fertile mucus throughout the cycle.**

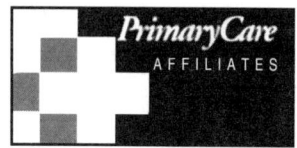

Vanessa M. Britto, M.D.

As a primary care physician in a women's health practice, I spend a substantial amount of time advising patients in preconceptual counseling. Many of my patients are educating themselves about healthy choices in family planning and ask about the possibility of gender selection. Theresa Hebert, in her book <u>Special Deliveries</u>, looks at this provocative issue in a very fascinating way. I look forward to recommending it to future parents as a wonderful alternative to "flipping a coin"!

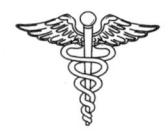

Vanessa M. Britto, M.D.
Internal Medicine

1300 Belmont Street, Brockton, Massachusetts 02401

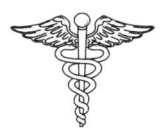

I have been a pediatric nurse for twenty-five years and was truly fascinated with your book *"Special Deliveries."* The idea of being able to choose the sex of a baby is a dream come true for many of the mothers I converse with.

Prior to my present job, I worked in the delivery room, hospital nursery and the obstetrics department. It has been my experience that, while many moms seem to have no particular preference for their first child, they usually will admit to secretly hoping for the opposite gender for their next baby. This book will give those with a preference the understanding that will be of great help in conceiving the preferred gender of a very precious little one.

It will be my pleasure to recommend *"Special Deliveries"* to all those moms and dads who are searching for the right method to help increase their gender selection.

Beverly J. DeMoranville, LPN
pediatric nurse
Massachusetts

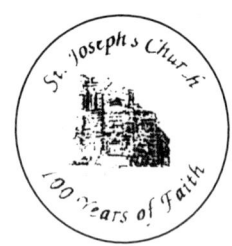

Saint Joseph's Parish
19 Kilmer Avenue
Taunton, MA 02780

Is it moral?

Yes. There are no restrictions to how a woman may go about planning the gender of her baby. The *"Special Deliveries"* method is a natural form of gender selection and it does not interfere in the conception process. Matter of fact, I find this study and method most interesting. I will certainly recommend Theresa Hebert's book to any woman who is searching in this area of life.

Sister Beth Mahoney

Sister Beth Mahoney, csc
(Congregation Sainte Croix)
Formerly Pastoral Assistant of
Saint Joseph's Parish
Taunton, Massachusetts
Now serving in other countries
around the globe.

ACKNOWLEDGEMENTS

I could not have started to bring new life into this world if it weren't for the life that my parents gave to me. Thank you Ma and Dad for all you have done for me throughout the years, and thanks for giving me my forever friends, my sister Marie and my brother Ray. Much gratitude to all of you for always being there for my family and me.

A special thanks to my grandmother who is the foundation of our family and our values.

To my husband, Glen, don't think I do not notice all that you do for our children and me. You are a wonderful husband and father.

"Special Deliveries" could not have been possible without special lifetime friends like David & Susan Kawa, Ray & Lynne Ducharme, Stan & Marie Pawlowski, Bruce Hebert, Jeannie & Dennis Hebert, Carol Ingram, and Bev & Lee DeMoranville. I extend my deepest appreciation for your constant support in all my endeavors.

To my nephews Nathan, Nick and Paul, you are each so unique and dear to me. I am very proud of what you have already accomplished in your young lives. Lastly to my niece, Rachel Elizabeth, you will always be a very *"Special Delivery"* to me!

"For the past 15 years, I have been researching the subject of gender selection and working on this book. My goal has always been the same: to share this information with others and let them know they have a safe, easy, natural alternative to the gender selection of their baby. By making others aware of the availability of this information they can then make their own educated decisions."

Theresa Hebert
Author

TABLE OF CONTENTS

PREFACE

"Special Deliveries" shows you how to improve your chances of having a baby boy or a girl by following a few safe and simple suggestions supported by scientific research, religions and doctors. **This book provides a precisely written, concise explanation with instructions and illustrations which are safe, easy-to-follow and natural.**

INTRODUCTION

I

HOW TO CHOOSE

A BIG OR GIRL BOY

I INTRODUCTION

When I was expecting, in particular my second and third children, I was convinced that people really do care whether their child will be a boy or girl. All I heard was, "I bet you want a girl" or "Wouldn't it be great if you had a girl this time" and, of course, the very popular, "Are you trying for a girl?" Before we had considered having our children, I had minimal knowledge of methods to conceive a boy or girl baby. So I started to search for more written material on this subject.

This book will try to explain that, indeed, there are no completely fool-proof methods to achieve the desired results, but there are ways to better your chances of having a baby of the gender of your choice. Having kept extensive records for each of my three pregnancies, I was convinced that these methods proved positive for me, and would work for anyone. With a little patience and effort, any couple could better their chances of influencing the gender of their baby. This is when I decided to take the time to write this book. I read book after book, spent every day in the library or local book stores and every book contradicted the one before.

Whether you're having your first child, or are planning to have another, you can increase the probability of conceiving the offspring of your choice by following a few simple suggestions described in this book.

THE RESEARCH

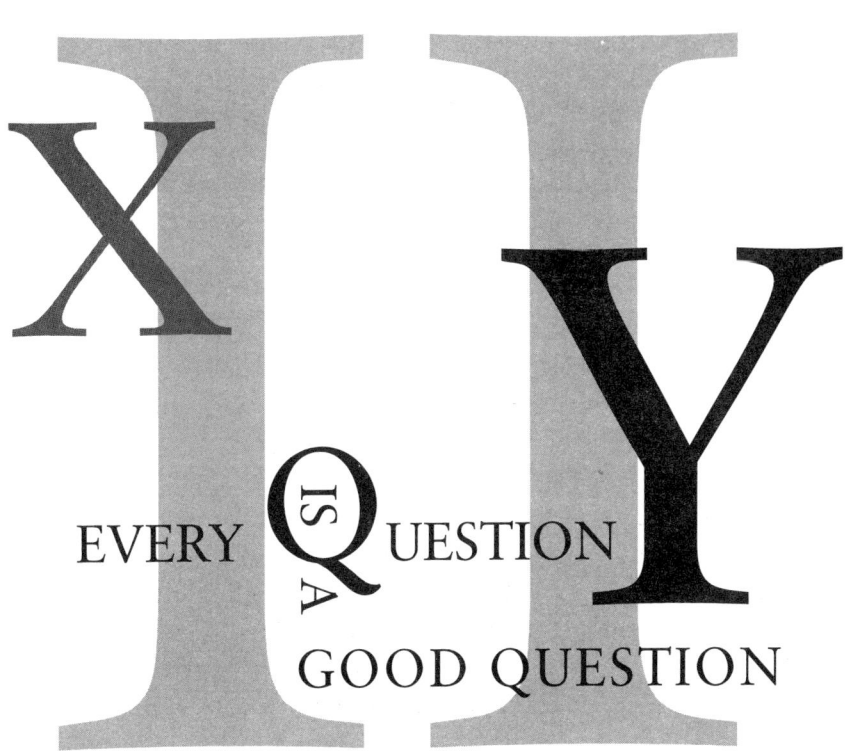

II

EVERY QUESTION IS A GOOD QUESTION

II   RESEARCH

During my extensive research, I found suggestions of all kinds. I read that if the father-to-be consumed large quantities of coffee (caffeine), " *it could impart some extra speed for the male producing sperm.*"[1], thus causing the conception of a boy. I also read that by douching with vinegar, a woman could increase her chances of having a girl. Also, positioning during relations supposedly could make a difference and even what you ate the day before.

In parts of the world it was said, long ago, that the man would bite his partner's right ear if he wanted a son, and her left ear for a daughter. But the best one was the Greek belief that the gender of the child is determined by the *"stronger"* or *"wiser"* of the two partners. I thought most of these myths sounded ludicrous and did not take them seriously.

Myth also would have us believe that men who wear tight fitting clothing or tight fitting shorts tend to have more girls. It is said that men who work near heat, toxic chemicals or certain drugs or on a job that might cause psychological stress, tend to have lower sperm counts which would increase their chances for a girl baby.

Despite all of the claims, myths and superstitions, all of my research indicated that the timing of a woman's ovulation is of primary importance regarding the selection of the gender of your baby.

"Timing is not just one of the elements you need to adhere to: it is the element that is most important. You can dispense with everything else and still have a good chance of succeeding if your timing is right."

So I read, researched and questioned more on the timing of a woman's ovulation, and practiced taking my basal body temperature (BBT) every morning as an indicator. This is known as the Temperature Method, as shown on *Figure 1*, illustrated on page 25. It is completely safe and very easy. The inconvenience seemed to be well worth the trouble. A BBT Thermometer can be purchased at any pharmacy or drugstore. If you prefer an ear or a regular digital thermometer, you may use it for an easier read. Whatever you plan to use, be consistent and use the same device each time.

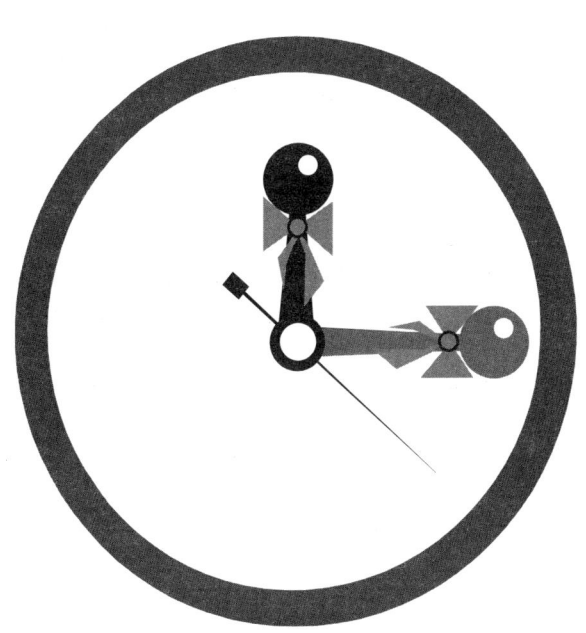

FIGURE 1: BASAL BODY TEMPERATURE INSTRUCTIONS

1. Fill in the dates across the top of the chart in advance. This will help you to remember to record your temperature each and every day.

2. Every morning, immediately after you awaken, place the basal body thermometer under your tongue and leave it in place for a full five minutes. (Please note: Some newer thermometers take as little as one minute to give you an accurate reading.) Readings should be taken at the same time every day whenever possible. But the time is not as important as the fact that you haven't risen out of bed and moved around. Do not eat, drink or smoke before taking your temperature.

3. Record the temperature reading on the chart by placing a dot on the appropriate horizontal line in the column beneath the date. If you miss a day, leave a blank column. Connect the points with a straight line.

4. Any events which could affect your temperature should be written in next to each point. These include: a cold, infection, insomnia or variation in sleep schedule, unusual stress and/or medications.

5. In the boxes provided at the top of the chart, check off the days on which you have sexual relations.

6. Check off the days of your menstrual period in the appropriate boxes at the top of the chart. If you are having menstrual periods, the first day of your menstrual flow is considered day 1 of your cycle; in this case, start a new chart on this day. If you are not having menstrual periods, complete one chart fully before starting the next.

FIGURE 1: BASAL BODY TEMPERATURE INSTRUCTIONS

MONTH/DAY																						

RELATIONS

MENSTRUAL CYCLE

MEDICATION

CYCLE

OVULATION

99.0
.9
.8
.7
.6
.5
.4
.3
.2
.1
98.0
.9
.8
.7
.6
.5
.4
.3
.2
.1
97.0

The very first time we tried conceiving we were successful. Our first son, Alex, was conceived exactly on the day of ovulation, charted by the BBT methods.

When I attempted to conceive my second child, Brent, I kept my BBT charts, acted on the results and tried for another son. We thought that having a brother for our first son would be great. At the time, we planned to have only two children, as we thought they would have more in common growing up together.

When my husband Glen and I decided to have a third child, we thought it would be nice to have a daughter. I used the Temperature Method and a home ovulation predictor test, followed the methods described in this book, and gave birth to our daughter, Arielle Elena.

Home ovulation predictor tests are available at any pharmacy or drugstore and they allow a woman to predict her ovulation time with a high degree of accuracy. It is especially helpful for women, like myself, who have irregular cycles (my menstrual cycle has ranged from 28 to 47 days). The use of the Temperature Method together with the home ovulation predictor test makes the timing of a woman's ovulation more accurate than either method used alone.

Obviously, if someone as irregular as myself can time ovulation, then it should be much easier for a woman that has a regular cycle (i.e. 28 days). Regularity does not affect the results, it just makes the job that much easier. Note that women who have regular 28 day cycles are likely to ovulate in the middle of their cycles, thus approximately on day 14.

Most couples planning to have a child know that having relations with their partner around the time of the woman's ovulation will likely lead to conception. Medical researchers have found that the closer a woman times intercourse with ovulation, the better the couple's chances are of conceiving a boy.

"The faster, male producing sperm will be most likely to reach the egg first and fertilize it when intercourse occurs at or near the time of ovulation, when the physiological secretions are most alkaline and thus most favorable for sperm penetration".[1]

For example, on my first pregnancy, I ovulated on day 19, had relations right on that day, and delivered a baby boy. With my second pregnancy, I had taken my temperature for months prior to conceiving. On the month that I conceived, I recorded ovulation on the 17th day of my cycle, also the day of relations, whereby eight months and 28 days later, we had our second son.

I was thrilled to deliver sons on my first two pregnancies. But when my husband and I decided to have a third child, we honestly thought that if this were to be our last child, it would be nice if the boys had a baby sister. And yes, wouldn't it be nice to have a daughter.

So, I researched even more about choosing the gender of my baby before conceiving. Past experience with my doctor seemed to indicate that he didn't give much credence to the idea that timing could be a factor in determining the baby's gender, but he was quite interested in what I had discovered. **I knew in my heart that I truly wanted another baby, no matter which gender it would be. The most important thing to me was to have a healthy baby.** I was very lucky to have two beautiful, healthy boys; couldn't we try to have a healthy girl this time?

HOW TO GET STARTED

RECORD YOUR FINDINGS

98.2°

98.6°

III
HOW TO GET STARTED

Before you attempt to conceive, spend a few months practicing timing your ovulation by taking your basal body temperature (BBT) every morning **before you rise out of bed.** Chart and graph your findings as described in Figure 1. (See page 25.) Additional blank charts are located on pages 103 & 105 for your personal use. Your gynecologist's office can provide you with any additional charts you will need. If you call ahead, you can make an appointment with the nurse specifically to explain and show you firsthand how the Temperature Method is done. You can even buy a regular digital or ear thermometer, available at any pharmacy or drugstore, to make your BBT easier to read.

Medical research suggests that the ovulation usually occurs right before the rise in temperature after the last low drop in temperature.

"Almost all women that keep accurate charts find that their BBT's are noticeably lower before ovulation than they are after ovulation, reflecting the overall phases of the cycle. Temperatures prior to ovulation are usually, but not always, somewhere between 97.4 and 97.8 (degrees Fahrenheit). After ovulation, the temperature increases usually by four-tenths to a full degree in a single day. Then it tends to stay high, almost always above 98 degrees, though it can still dip up and down a bit. In the post ovulatory phase of the cycle, the BBT typically lingers between 98.2 and 98.6 degrees." [1]

Once the temperature goes up and stays high, you can be sure that the ovulation has already taken place. Figure 1, illustrated on page 25, is an example of my personal chart. Note that the last low temperature before the sudden rise in temperature shows that the ovulation occurred on day 16. I was also expecting my period on day 30 which was 14 days after ovulation, further evidence that the BBT peak correctly indicated ovulation.

After a few months of practicing, I suggest a minimum of 6, 9 , 12 or more, you will probably begin to notice a pattern in your ovulation. Menstruation usually occurs some constant number of days after ovulation. You can use this to check your charted ovulation cycle. For example: if on your first BBT chart, you menstruate on the 14th day after the indicated ovulation, check that the subsequent charts show the same 14 day interval.

Once you are feeling confident with the Temperature Method for predicting ovulation, it is time to purchase a home predictor kit, preferably the kind that tells you at least 24 to 36 hours in advance when you'll be ovulating. These kits are available at most pharmacies and drugstores.

The home ovulation predictor chart in Figure 2, depicted on page 33, shows that when the color turns the deepest, it indicates a rise in the level of Luteinizing Hormone (LH).

Ovulation should occur within 24 to 36 hours of your first color increase. In my case, shown in Figure 2, the color increase occurred on day 15, which would indicate that ovulation would be on the following day: day 16. This is confirmed by the BBT chart in Figure 1, which indicated ovulation on the day before the peak.

Figure 2: Home Ovulation Predictor Chart Example

(see Figure 2 on opposite page)

Using the Temperature Method and the home ovulation predictor test, you can now time your relations with respect to ovulation, in order to influence the gender of the conceived baby. If you're trying for a girl, you should stop having relations at least 48 hours prior to ovulation. It's best to try 2 to 3 days before, to be on the safe side. If, on the other hand, you're trying for a boy, concentrate relations on the day of ovulation **only.**

My husband and I followed this method, ceased having relations prior to ovulation and successfully conceived a girl. Remember that the X (female) sperm are heartier than the Y (male) sperm, and are more resistant to various forms of stress, while the Y sperm are quicker. If you are going to become pregnant, and you have ceased relations 2 to 3 days prior to ovulation, it's more likely that the larger, more resistant X sperm will still be lurking high up in the fallopian tubes, waiting to fertilize the egg when it appears.

FIGURE 2: HOME OVULATION PREDICTION CHART-EXAMPLE

Date of First Test 1-July	Days After Your Period Began		Test Results (SHADING)		
	5				
	⑥				
	7				
	8				
	⑨	Days 5			
	⑩	Prior 4			
	⑪	3			
	⑫	2			
1ST	13	✖			
2ND	⑭	✖			
3RD	15			✖	
4TH	16	OV →	✖		
5TH	17				
	18				
	19				
	20				
	21				
	22				
	23				
	24				
	25				
	26				
	27				
	28				

"If you have relations between 48 and 96 hours before ovulation, your chances of having a girl are greater." 1

" In a case where odd factors were at work: a truck driver who operated on a regular schedule that allowed him to be home only at certain times, and thus, never had relations with his wife after the 12th day of her cycle (when she regularly ovulated on day 14) this couple had three girls." 1

If scheduling your pregnancy for a certain time of year is important, you can practice these charting and prediction methods for months before actually conceiving.

Between taking your temperature and the home ovulation prediction test, you'll have two easy and safe ways of predicting the time you ovulate. Some, but not all women, notice a twinge of cramping at the time of ovulation: this is yet another indicator known as the **Mittelschmerz Method**. Mittelschmerz is a German word referring to the middle of the menstrual cycle and a pain that is felt at the time of ovulation in the lower abdomen on the right side.

THE BOTTOM LINE

BOY

FEMALE

GIRL

MALE

IV

III
THE BOTTOM LINE

A. To increase your chances of conceiving a girl

You may have intercourse daily from the time your period ceases to 2-3 days prior to ovulation and then again only after 6 or more days after ovulation. Remember, you should abstain completely for the 6 day period after ovulation, since it is possible that intercourse during that time could stimulate female secretions that might favor another male producing sperm.

" *The larger and more resistant female producing sperm will be most likely to fertilize the egg when intercourse takes place at least two days in advance of ovulation, when the secretions are still more acidic, and thus more likely to eliminate the less resistant Y sperm*". [1]

B. To increase your chances of conceiving a boy

Abstain from intercourse for at least 4 days prior to ovulation. Then have intercourse only on the exact day of ovulation and then abstain for at least 6 days afterwards. When you resume, use a condom to assure that you conceived when you planned to. During the abstinence period prior to ovulation, intercourse is not advisable (for the same reasons mentioned earlier).

" *There is some evidence now to indicate that intercourse at the exact time of ovulation (14 days before the onset of the next menstrual period) is more likely to produce a male infant.*" [2]

MY
PERSONAL & EXPERIENCE

KNOWLEDGE

SUCCESS

HOPE

V

V

MY PERSONAL EXPERIENCE

When trying for my third child, I knew from the research I had calculated using BBT charting and the home ovulation predictor test, that my best chance to conceive a girl was at least two days prior to ovulation. I ovulated on day 16 and the intercourse that resulted in the conception of our daughter happened on day 14.

For the first few months I was trying to get pregnant, my husband and I ceased having relations three days prior to ovulation, just to be on the safe side.

" The idea is to time intercourse well in advance of ovulation, as far in advance as possible to begin with, but not so far as to completely rule out the chance of conceiving at all." [3]

When I did not get pregnant, we moved having relations up two days before ovulation. It took only two months, at two days prior, to become pregnant. Of course this happened after several months of charting and becoming familiar with my ovulation cycle. I only needed two home ovulation predictor tests.

Six weeks before I had my daughter, I had a second routine ultrasound test done. The technician predicted it was a girl, but realizing that they are not always accurate in their predictions, my husband and I kept the news to ourselves. Knowing that we had timed it according to the methods I have explained, gave us more confidence that the technician was right.

Since having our children, I have wanted to share my happiness and help others experience the same success. It is my contention that most people really do hope for a baby of one gender over the other. Maybe not so frequently if it is their first child, but more so on their second or third. Now when I hear someone ask an expectant mother, " *What are you hoping for?*", I think to myself, *"Why not supplement that hope with a little knowledge?"* This method is easy, safe and natural.

While some say that couples should just be content to have healthy children and of course that should be everyone's top priority, it does not change the fact that couples everywhere continue to long for the opposite gender. I have received numerous phone calls and letters of appreciation from couples thanking me for understanding their desires and reiterating what they feel is a **natural human desire**, which is timeless and universal! These letters continue to confirm the desire that people have for **both genders.** I continue to hear from grandparents as well, who want the book for their children and ask, *"Where was your book when I was having children?"*

A grandmother from Kansas called in October of 1997 to say: "I used your method in theory 27 years ago. I had 4 girls, used this method of timing and completed our family with our son Patrick, who was born on June 15, 1970. Patrick also used the method himself after having had 1 girl and his son Alex was born on February 28, 1995.

*A mother holds
her children's hands
for awhile...
their hearts forever.*

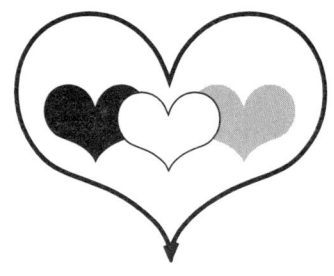

FOR YOUR
INFORMATION

NATURAL HUMAN

UNIVERSAL TIMELESS

BALANCE

VI

DESIRE

VI
FOR YOUR INFORMATION

My reason for writing this book is simple. There seems to be universal experience among couples bearing their first child: people automatically assume they will want the opposite sex the second time around. Comments abound to that effect, and, of course, it gets worse when they have two, three or even more children of the same gender.

Following the simple procedure described in this book, my husband and I conceived the baby of our choice not once, but THREE TIMES!! It was all accomplished without artificial means: simply with a little patience and some knowledge and understanding of the human body. With a little motivation, I truly believe it can work for you, too, as it has for people all over the globe. (See *"Special Deliveries"* testimonials on pages 76-91.)

Remember, if you want something badly enough, it's worth putting some time and effort toward achieving your goal. Time has taught us nothing in life comes easy. If you are thinking that it is too much trouble to follow these methods, just let God decide. Remember, **God is deciding** and He also gave us the free will to make use of the knowledge provided to us by our peers and predecessors. I believe you can and should use that free will to make yourself happier and more content. Indeed God is the ultimate decision maker in all our lives!!

"Special Deliveries" surveys, testimonials, letters and daily phone calls all continue to strengthen the belief that there is a **genuine balance of desire for both genders.** As social and economic constraints continue to escalate throughout the world, I truly believe this book will help people fulfill their prayers, wishes, hopes and dreams for their complete and happy family.

In case this is of interest to you, the Catholic Church, through Monsignor H. Currant, Director of the Family Bureau for the Archdiocese of New York, has said that the church has no objections to gender selections. *"As long as the intent of these efforts is not to prevent conception."*

I found that most religions incorporate this natural form of gender selection into their family planning methods.

LETTERS FROM THE MEDIA

COMMUNICATE

EDUCATE

PRODUCERS

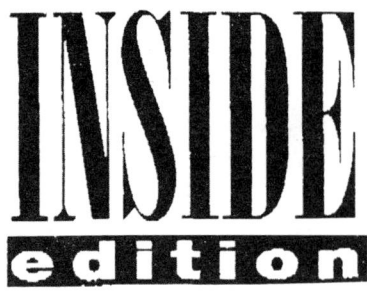

September 22, 1997

"Special Deliveries"
67 South Crane Ave.
Taunton, MA 02780

Attention: Theresa Hebert

Dear Theresa:

Just wanted to drop you a note to thank you again for your hospitality and kindness while we were there shooting the story on "Special Deliveries". I know I speak for Dave and Joe when I say we really had a wonderful day and truly enjoyed spending time with you and your family.

The story isn't scheduled as of yet, but I will keep you posted on the progress. Please stay in touch and happy belated birthday!

Gary Wynn
PRODUCER

Segment aired in October 1997

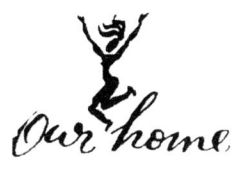

Our home,

August 29, 1997

"Special Deliveries"
67 South Crane Ave.
Taunton, MA 02780

Attention:Theresa Hebert

Dear Theresa:

On behalf of all of us at OUR HOME, thank you so much for taking the time out of your busy schedule to appear on our show. You were a wonderful guest on the air and also a pleasure to work with. We think the segment was worthwhile and informative and appreciate your input and enthusiasm. It was great to work with you. We hope your trip back was pleasant.

We are so appreciative of the wonderful gifts that you brought. It was so nice of you. We know we'll enjoy them.

We hope that you feel that we covered all of the important information that needed to be covered. We'll call you with an airdate as soon as we get word.

Sincerely,

Shari Lampert
Producer

Kristin Cosover
Associate
Producer

lifetime studios 34-12 36th street   astoria, ny 11106
SEGMENT AIRED IN OCTOBER OF 1997

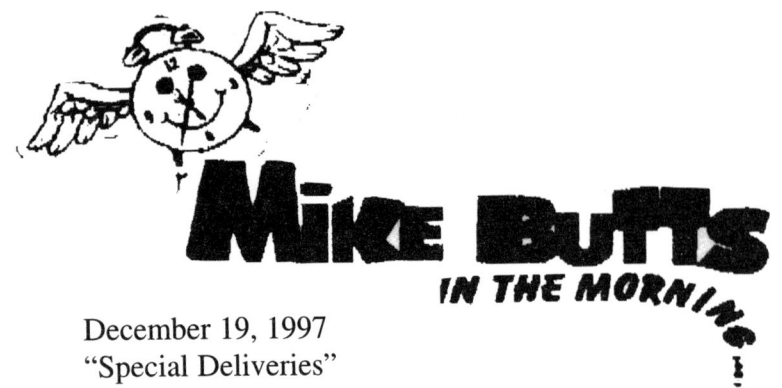

December 19, 1997
"Special Deliveries"
67 South Crane Ave.
Taunton, MA 02780

Attention: Theresa Hebert

Dear Theresa:

As I celebrate my 5th year with 92 PRO FM today, I wanted to thank you for the appearances you've made on my morning show and the people you have helped, my listeners.

With all the babies that you've helped plan, I'm surprised the Mayor up there doesn't officially change the name of the street you live on, Crane, to "STORK" Avenue.

You certainly have developed a way to help people plan their family and my listeners love talking with you. I hope you'll come back and see us again and I wish you all the best in 1998!

Love Always,

MIKE BUTTS "IN THE MORNING"
5:30-10AM
92 PRO-FM
PROVIDENCE
CITADEL COMMUNICATIONS CORPORATION

KDWB

"Special Deliveries"
67 South Crane Ave.
Taunton, MA 02780
Attention: Theresa Hebert

Dear Theresa:

Just a note to thank you for being on our radio show. You are a fabulous, funny, informative and entertaining guest. Our listeners were very interested in knowing that they themselves can play an active role in pre-planning the gender of their baby. There was much interest surrounding the topic of your book.

We thoroughly enjoyed having you as a guest on our radio show, both in 1996 and 1997. You were a wonderful guest and I believe a kind and generous person as well. You are an inspiration and we can't wait to have you back again. Best wishes for the new book and to you for the New Year.

Sincerely,

"Dave Ryan in the Morning Show"
100 N. Sixth Street
Suite 306C
Minneapolis, Minnesota 55403
(612)340-9000

Dave Ryan
KDWB Radio
"1996 Marconi Award Winner"

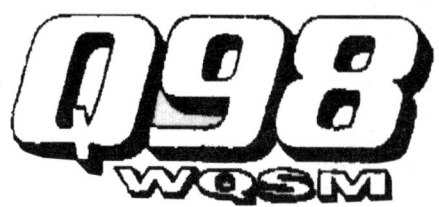

"Special Deliveries"
67 South Crane Ave.
Taunton, MA 02780

Attention: Theresa Hebert

Dear Theresa:

Thank you for being on our show, Q98's "Morning Palooza", to talk about "Special Deliveries". The show was a huge success and we received lots of calls from both men and women, not only during the show, but after the show as well.

There seem to be a lot of people who would like to choose the sex of their child/children and "Special Deliveries" gives them the information they need.

We were thrilled to hear that your book has been so successful and that you are now printing a new edition.

We and our listeners are really looking forward to speaking to you again on the show next month.

Wishing you every success for the future

With Best Wishes,
Q98's Morning Palooza

ON BEHALF OF RICK JENSEN,
DAVID JAMES, ZELLY RESTORICK-LOPEZ

1009 DRAYTON RD. * P.O. BOX 35297 * FAYETTEVILLE, NC 28303
(910) 864-5222 * FAX (910) 864-3065
WQSM-FM/ 100,000 WATTS

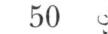

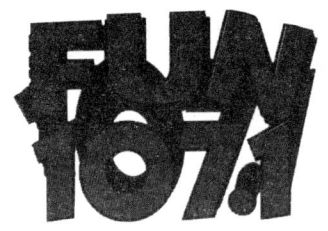

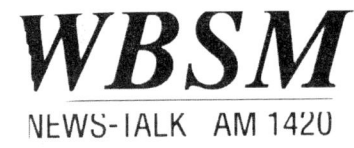

NEWS-TALK   AM 1420

"Special Deliveries"
67 South Crane Ave.
Taunton, MA 02780

Attention: Theresa Hebert

Theresa has been a guest on the "Fun Morning Crew" on numerous occasions and is a tremendous draw every time. She is knowledgeable, witty and passionate about her work. She truly believes in educating people and is willing to share her own personal experience in order to help others.

She is a welcomed guest on our morning show today and always!

Sincerely,

JR & SHARON
"THE FUN MORNING CREW"

22 SCONTIOUT NECK ROAD * FAIRHAVEN, MASSACHUSETTS 02719
FAX: 508-999-1420 * FM * 508-999-5590 * AM * 508-9991787

"Special Deliveries"
67 South Crane Ave.
Taunton, MA 02780

Attention: Theresa Hebert

I first met Theresa several years ago and immediately knew she was bound for great things. She is one of the most dynamic people I've ever met.

As a guest on "For Women Only" she reached out to couples everywhere by sharing not only her research in "Special Deliveries", but sharing her personal experience. She is an interviewer's dream. She knows what she is talking about and is brilliant in spreading her message.

Theresa Hebert is a true pro!

I consider her to be a friend and a role model for people everywhere. I wish her nothing but the best.

Sincerely,

SHARON FORGERAN
ABC 6 HEALTH CONTRIBUTOR

MOM'S TALK

P.O. BOX 466 MT. AIRY, MD 21771

"Special Deliveries"
67 South Crane Ave.
Taunton, MA 02780

Attention: Theresa Hebert

We heard about your book "Special Deliveries" through CNN and we are looking forward to having you as a guest on our show in 1998 to discuss your book.

We feel that both stay-at-home and working Moms are being overlooked in society today. There are not enough resources out there for Moms to turn where they can get immediate feedback. That's where we come in! MOM'S TALK is a weekly, live call in radio talk show on WFMD AM 930 in Frederick, Maryland. Our show provides a nonthreatening forum for Moms to call in or write with their ideas, suggestions, problems, or just to vent their daily frustrations.

We have a lot of exciting and fun things planned for MOM'S TALK in 1998. We hope to obtain corporate sponsorship for our show and take our show nationwide so that we can reach every Mom in the country. MOM'S TALK- an idea whose time has come!

Sincerely,

Lynne

LYNNE   KATHLEEN   BARBI

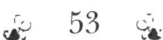

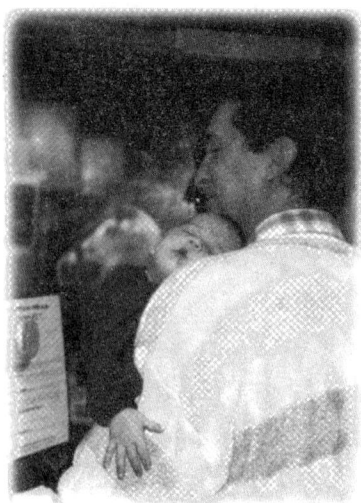

"Ray to the Rescue"
My brother Ray calming a *"Special Deliveries"* baby during the live radio show

Kristen Ciacciarelli (*"Special Deliveries" testimonial & 92 PRO-FM listener*)

Mike Butts, *D.J., 92 PRO-FM*

Theresa Hebert, *Author*

Lisa Butts, *D.J., 92 PRO-FM*

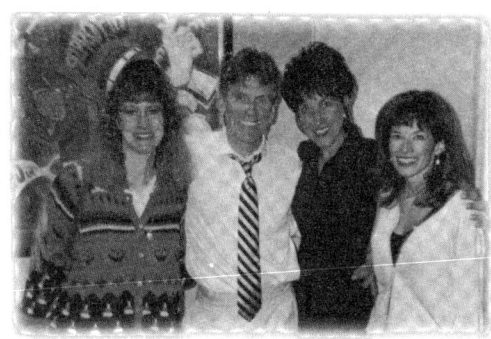

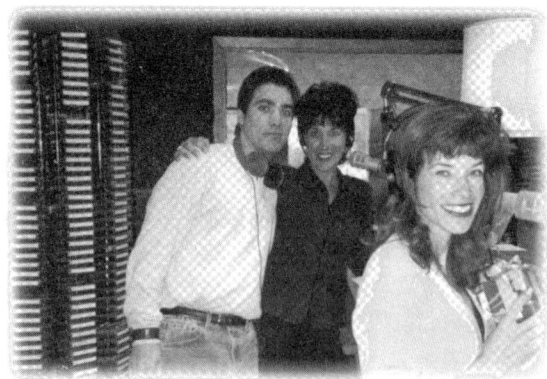

While doing live radio show on 92 PRO-FM
"Rockin Joe Hebert"
Theresa Hebert
Lisa Butts

 54 ﹒ஃ

SPECIAL DELIVERIES
UPDATE

On July 10, 1996, I appeared on my first live radio show. It was in-studio at 92 Pro-FM in Providence, Rhode Island with Mike and Lisa Butts, "Rockin Joe Hebert" and friends. Since that time I have appeared on more than 350 radio interviews worldwide all over the United States and as far away as Australia and Alaska. It is true that you never forget about things that you do first - your first kiss, first love, first radio show. Mike and Lisa Butts will always hold a special place in my heart. They are the most generous, thoughtful, and funniest D.J.'s on radio. Along with "Rockin Joe" and friends they continue to get me up each morning, laughing and with a smile on my face. Then I'm ready to do my radio shows and consultations with people from around the globe. So, if you live in the Southern New England area or are just here for a visit, keep your radio dial on 92 Pro-FM, you'll be glad you did.

My appearance on national television came before radio. My most recent national television appearances include **Lifetime Television for Women**, **Inside Edition**, and **CNN**. Some of my past goals are now being realized. This method of natural family planning is offered as a choice by doctors, and supported by religions across the country.

In April of 1996, a gentleman from Wisconsin, originally from Yugoslavia, called me to tell me of his friend in Yugoslavia who just had his ninth child, a boy after eight girls. That story exemplifies the natural human desire that all couples experience. The man from Wisconsin went on to say, " I have two daughters and I love them dearly. However, I don't want six or seven more before I have a son. My wife and I plan on using *'Special Deliveries'.*"

SPECIAL DELIVERIES MOTTO

" KNOW WHAT YOU WANT AND LOVE WHAT YOU GET. ANY BABY IS THE RIGHT BABY... YOUR BABY!"

If you are planning to conceive a child and would lovingly welcome any baby into your home there is a way to increase your chances of having a daughter after four wonderful sons, or a son after two beautiful daughters. There is absolutely no harm in trying this safe, easy, non-invasive, natural way.

It is my belief that God is the ultimate decision maker in all our lives. We are on this earth to help and learn from each other. Each generation builds on the one before it and each one moves us toward greater control of our own lives. "God helps those who help themselves".

Do you know what the most often asked question of expectant mothers is besides, "How are you feeling?" and "Would you like another pickle with your ice cream?" Of course it's: "What are you hoping for, a baby boy or girl?" Isn't it natural for a couple who has four boys at home and expecting again, to hope for a girl this time? So you don't have to stand on your head and eat a bunch of bananas while wearing pink socks to have a girl! You can do that if it happens to be your preference, but isn't it easier to get your timing right? Timing is everything.

I am so happy when I'm on a radio show and people call in and say things like, " Theresa, I used your book back in 1992 and I wanted a boy and then two girls and it worked for me each time. I have friends and family members who have also used it successfully." In September of 1996 while interviewing on a live radio show in Canada, the first caller was a doctor calling to say, "Some of my patients have your book. I had the opportunity to read it and I think you are providing a great service to mankind.
KEEP UP THE GOOD WORK!"

Another of my goals is to have doctors everywhere offer this method in theory to their patients. At least give them their options, let them know they have this natural choice. Then let them make the best decision for themselves.

When a woman goes to her OB-GYN's office and asks for a way to increase her chances of having either a baby boy or girl before her next pregnancy she now has some options. More doctors are referring their patients to either laboratory procedures as an alternative or "*Special Deliveries*", as a safe, easy, natural method that is a moral, ethical and a financial solution to your planned family. Finally, people are becoming educated and aware that they have a choice. After all, the power of choice is a God-given attribute.

I have found in the past that some doctors and certain people criticize concepts that they don't understand. Sometimes they are just unwilling to accept a different approach to an uncommon subject. Upon reading this book they realize there is absolutely no harm to this method and they tend to make comments like, "Wow, this makes so much sense, why didn't anyone tell me this before?" Well, the truth is, similar information has been available for many years, yet people are still unaware they have the power to educate themselves. They can become more knowledgeable about their own bodies and influence the chance of gender selection. Remember, it is as simple as timing to increase your chances of a baby boy or girl rather than just timing to conceive a child. I have to say it pleases me greatly when someone calls to say "I've read several books on this subject, searched the Internet and the library and have found your book to be the simplest to follow!" This is precisely why I wrote this book, to give people a simpler approach.

I can't tell you how gratifying it is and what a real sense of fulfillment I receive in sharing this information to help others pursue their happiness. People contact me daily to tell me their dreams and compelling stories of longing for a baby boy or baby girl. There are just as many scenarios of the perfect family as there are people in the world. Many women have health issues and concerns that often restrict their child bearing possibilities. For example, girl babies tend to carry the gene for hemophilia, while boy babies contract the disease itself. (Hemophilia is a hereditary disorder in which the blood fails to clot normally, causing prolonged bleeding from even minor injuries.) Others include specific hereditary chromosome deficiencies. Every couple wants to bring a healthy baby into the world. Some couples have children from a previous relationship and would like to extend their family. One of my main goals is to help alleviate the guilt that people have had in the past regarding gender selection and let them know that what they are feeling is completely natural and that the emotions they are expressing are universal and timeless. People around the world call me and attest to those feelings everyday. Most people express their feelings of wanting to experience what it's like to have both a son and a daughter.

"Special Deliveries" method is based on the theory that it is not just the male that determines the gender of the baby. The male and female both play a part in determining the gender. We know that the man contributes the sex chromosomes (XX for female and XY for male), but some are still unaware that it is actually the environment in a woman's body at the time of relations that will favor either the X female producing sperm or the Y male producing sperm.

Two, three or four days prior to ovulation a woman's physiological secretions are more acidic, thus favoring the female producing sperm. The stronger, hardier X female producing sperm are able to survive and last longer in the acidic environment. So, if a woman has relations days prior and then ceases and conceives, it is likely the X female producing sperm will be lurking high up in the fallopian tubes waiting to fertilize the egg. On the other hand, if relations occur as close as possible to ovulation, on the day of ovulation or just hours before ovulation when the woman's physiological secretions are more alkaline, this will favor the Y male producing sperm that are smaller, quicker and swim faster to reach the egg. Fertilization is possible due to the alkaline environment, which is more conducive to the Y male producing sperm. So, men, stop blaming yourself for producing only one gender, it really does take two. I'm always thrilled when a person calls to say, "I read your book and then my partner read it and then we read it together."

BE PATIENT!

Sometimes women consult with me and feel unsure of their cycles and when they are ovulating. They may say, "I think I am ovulating on this particular day, but I'm not sure." I usually recommend that they continue to chart their cycles for a few more months and then 6, 9 or 12 months later they call me again and very confidently say, " I know I'm ovulating on this day". That is when you are ready to go ahead and try for the gender of your choice. **I want to strongly stress that you now have the information you need to make it possible to conceive either a boy or girl baby. But what you personally need to add to this equation is patience. Take your time!** For all good things come to those who wait. I have women who call me and say, "I just read your book and I'd like to try to get pregnant next month." It's a wonderful thing to advise her to wait and have her call me many months later to thank me because she just had a baby girl after four boys. **Stop and Think**- I suggest waiting at least 6 months or more, the more the better. Once you see a pattern of your own individual cycles, you will begin to feel when ovulation is occurring. <u>**Chart as long as you can for the most successful results.**</u>

For those of you that use a Home Ovulation Predictor Test Kit, make sure you use at least one as an experiment before using the kit when you are actually ready to try. Please read the instructions very carefully. Some kits will let you know 12-24 hours prior to ovulation, while others 24-48 hours or longer.

Make sure when you see a darker color change you realize the LH surge is happening. If you are trying for a boy, don't have relations right away. Make sure you wait at least 24 hours - 36 hours to be sure you are as close to ovulation as possible. On the other hand, if your hope is for a girl, when you see the color change, cease everything. DO NOT have relations because ovulation will be occurring anywhere between 12-48 hours. Again, read your instructions carefully.

Many people from all over the world have contacted and thanked me for sharing this information to help make it possible for them to have their desired child. Some women have made comments such as, "you're an angel" and "you're doing something very special". "I didn't even know what ovulation was or when it was happening to me until I read your book." For those of you who are still unsure...

Ovulation: is that time in a woman's cycle when a mature egg stored in the ovaries, breaks out and is then able to be fertilized by the sperm. Ovulation does not only occur on day 14, but rather a different day for each individual woman, depending on the length of her menstrual cycle.

A recent story on a well known magazine show interviewed a woman who chose artificial insemination. Unfortunately, she was given the wrong specimen sample, and was impregnated with someone other than her own husband's sperm and contracted the AIDS virus. This is just one example of why it is so important to weigh all your options and educate yourself to all the possible pros and cons.

A testimony from New York: Kim R. and her husband made an appointment to consult with a doctor they saw on a television program. His gender selection program included taking hormones or fertility drugs. Some fertility drugs such as Clomid can cause an increase in multiple births as well as an increase in the severity of migraine headaches. Each individual procedure is costly and not always successful the first time. This couple had two boys and desperately wanted to complete their family with a little girl. After considering their options, including the risks of side effects, they decided to use the *"Special Deliveries"* natural method. I am very happy to announce their daughter, Jenna Layne, was born on June 5th, 1997.

Something to consider: Fertility drugs have been known to cause multiple births. People usually assume they could have twins, triplets, even quadruplets. But, do they ever consider possibly having as many as seven children at once. It can and has happened!

FERTILE OR INFERTILE?

If you have waited the recommended time of 6, 9, 12 or more months charting, etc. (The Testing Period) before actually trying to conceive a child, try not to get discouraged when once you decide to actively try to conceive and you are confident you have pinpointed your day of ovulation you don't conceive right away. So, you know you're fertile, you time relations perfectly and you don't get pregnant. What's wrong?

So many couples call me discouraged when months pass and nothing happens. Keep in mind it is not as easy to conceive a child as one might think. When I began researching years ago, I remember thinking how amazing it was that anyone has children when you consider all the biologically intricate details that have to occur in order for conception to occur.

Not only do you have to get your timing accurate but, "the quality" of the egg is a factor as well as the quality of its migration through the fallopian tube, the quality of the sperm and its ability to get to and penetrate the egg, the readiness of the uterine lining to accept an embryo. All of these and more contribute to whether or not conception will occur to any given couple at any given time.

This is why it takes the average couple four to six months to get pregnant. Because the viability of a woman's eggs diminishes with age, it takes even longer when the woman is over 35. In fact, the odds of conceiving in any given month drop from 25 percent for the average twenty something couple, to about 5 percent among couples in which the woman is over 40. Don't get discouraged though. Many women in their forties go on to have beautifully healthy children. More and more women today are exercising and eating healthier than ever before which helps ensure a healthy pregnancy.

When To See A Fertility Doctor

If you are in your twenties and have no risk factors for infertility, wait at least a year before consulting a specialist. **Seek help sooner if:**

◆   You are over 35, since the viability of your eggs decreases as you near 40.

◆   You have a history of endometriosis, sexually transmitted disease or pelvic inflammatory disease - all common causes of infertility.

◆   You have erratic menstrual cycles - especially more than 35 days apart.

◆   You determine that you are not ovulating (based on the ovulation predictor kits or basal body temperature).

Be aware that it is a bad idea to jump the gun on fertility treatment. Clomiphene (Clomid), a popular ovulation enhancing drug, can dry up cervical fluid and make egg implantation difficult in women who do not truly need it. Fertility drugs should never be prescribed unless both partners have undergone thorough workups. And of course, let's not forget the possibility of multiple births once on fertility drugs. I know it is easier said than done, but try to be patient and let nature take its course.

Some of the Most Often Asked Questions

1. **How long in a woman's cycle is she actually fertile?**

    The woman's egg can only live up to 24 hours. However, two or more eggs may be released over a maximum of 24 hours. So, in a vacuum, a woman is only fertile for about a day or two. But the man's sperm can live up to five days, so the combined fertility of the two individuals is about a week.

2. **Do I have to wake up every day at the same time in order to take my temperature? I have other babies that keep me up!**

    No, although you should try to be as consistent as possible. In general, waking temperatures tend to creep up about two-tenths of a degree for every extra hour you sleep in. Thus, if you take it substantially later than usual, it may result in a reading that is outside the range of your usual pattern. If you wake up earlier than usual, you should take your temperature upon awakening, so long as you have had three hours of consecutive sleep.

3. **Do most women ovulate on day 14 of their cycle?**

    While most people assume the average women ovulates on day 14 of her cycle, the truth is the average woman is more irregular in her cycles than regular. So the answer is NO! The day of ovulation can vary among women as well as within each individual woman. However, once a woman ovulates, the time between ovulation and her menstruation is very consistent, almost always between 12 and 16 days. Within most individual women, this length of time generally doesn't change by more than a day or two. In other words, many women find once they ovulate that indeed they do regularly get their period 14 days later with an occasional variation of a day or two.

4.   WHAT IS MULTIPLE OVULATION?

Multiple ovulation is the release of two or more eggs in a single cycle. It occurs within 24 hours or less, after which no more eggs will be released until the following cycle. It is responsible for the birth of fraternal twins, as opposed to identical twins, which are the result of a single egg that divides after fertilization. Although this happens to many women naturally, it is a well known fact that fertility drugs increase the chances of multiple ovulations.

5.   HOW EXACTLY ARE FRATERNAL TWINS CONCEIVED? HOW WOULD THAT PROVE OR DISPROVE YOUR THEORY?

Fraternal twins (from two different eggs) are usually the same sex, which would support the idea that timing of relations is of critical importance in determining the sex of the baby. Since fraternal twins are conceived within 24 hours of each other, the conditions within the mother's reproductive tract are presumably the same for each conception. In the cases where the twins are boy and girl, they are both more than likely conceived on the borderline of two separate conditions be one acidic and the other closer to the alkaline environment.

6.   IF THIS METHOD OF TIMING TO CONCEIVE A BOY OR GIRL REALLY WORKS, WHY DON'T MORE DOCTORS TELL US ABOUT IT?

One of the most critical and mystifying reasons that people have rarely heard of it from their doctors is that doctors are seldom taught a comprehensive version of this scientific method in medical school. It is amazing to think that some men and women that I have had the pleasure to speak with over the years, have educated themselves and, in some cases, have more knowledge about a specific subject than some of their own doctors and gynecologists who are trained to be experts in female physiology. As I have said on numerous occasions, anyone can educate themselves in any subject they care deeply enough about.

6. (continued)

I can't tell you how many women who thought they were having trouble conceiving were told by some doctors to just have relations on day 14 and it will happen. When after educating herself she realizes she has never ovulated on day 14 but rather day 18 or 19. No wonder she didn't get pregnant. It wasn't a fertility problem, but rather an educational one.

Patients are now sharing this book with their doctors who have read it and agreed it is a natural alternative for some patients searching for a way to increase their chances of a boy or girl baby.

7. WHAT IS ENDOMETRIOSIS? CAN I GET PREGNANT IF I HAVE IT?

Endometriosis is one of the most widely diagnosed fertility problems. But take heed, there is help and women have gone from having successful surgeries to eliminate this problem to conception almost immediately with very normal healthy pregnancies and births. (See Douglass Testimonial from Florida, page 87).

Endometriosis is a prevalent disorder in which normal endometrial tissue like that which lines the uterus grows outside the uterus. This misplaced tissue may develop anywhere within the abdominal cavity, growing in small patches, larger nodules or within cysts in the ovary. The condition is highly unpredictable, because you could have a bad case and feel no pain or rather a mild case with excruciating pain. So any additional questions, ask your doctor, go for a check up.

8. IS IT TRUE THAT STANDING ON YOUR HEAD AIDS IN CONCEPTION?

You don't need to stand on your head for half an hour after relations in order to get pregnant! If you are timing relations at the most fertile time, 2-3 days prior to ovulation for a girl or the day of ovulation for a boy, the sperm will swim up through the cervical fluid rapidly, regardless of what position you are in. Remember, those of you trying for a girl need to be a little more patient and give it time. Those trying for a girl always risk the chance of getting impatient and thinking well maybe I just can't get pregnant with a girl and move it up a day, and voila become pregnant with a boy.

9. DO COUPLES WANT MORE BOYS OR GIRLS?

It has been my experience that just as many couples hope for girls as they do boys; it depends on what they already have. But the simple fact that there are boys and girls in the world make it a genuine, even balance.

"SPECIAL DELIVERIES"
Explanation of Benefits

"Special Deliveries" as seen on national T.V. is backed by scientific research. Proven effective, recommended by doctors, and supported by religious philosophies as a **safe, easy and natural** way to plan your family, *"Special Deliveries"* has testimonials all over the country and now in other parts of the world as well, since 1990.

"Special Deliveries" gives couples the information they desire in a simpler and more direct manner. It is easy to follow and gets right-to-the-point. You could spend years on research trying to decipher the information in other books or programs and years trying to figure out which methods to follow.

OR

Simplify your efforts with the *"Special Deliveries"* method that has and is currently helping countless couples everywhere achieve their desired results. This program has nothing to do with diet, positioning, drugs, or lab procedures, which makes this program a moral, ethical and financial solution to family planning. As any testimonial will tell you, *"Special Deliveries"* information is well worth any price for a lifetime of enjoyment with their child. *"Special Deliveries"* gives you an option to planning your family.

People everywhere continue to have children and will forever be looking for their Special Delivery. *"Special Deliveries"* gives couples the information to increase their chances of having either a son to carry on the family name or a daughter to complete their family. This program can be conveniently delivered right to your home and you are able to confer with the author herself through telephone, fax or other written consultations.

THE
BEST THING
TO
SPEND
ON
YOUR CHILD
IS
TIME

Some of our favorite family time spent together over the years has been reading together. When my children were small I always read to them. Now that they are older we read together. One of our favorite authors is Shel Silverstein, author of many poem and drawing books, intended to amuse all ages. Some of his titles include: "Where the Sidewalk Ends", "A Light In the Attic" and "Falling Up". We have many enjoyable hours, smiling, laughing and reading together. I'm sure you would agree, it is time well spent.

Here is a poem that my mother shared with me
when I was first expecting. I've since shared it with others
and now I gladly share it with you!!

THESE LAST FEW HOURS

Dee Dee McColl

It is important to me
    that I spend a part
    of the next few hours here
    alone with you in the darkness

You and I
    will never be this close again
    By morning
    you will be a tiny person
    all your own.

No longer the kicking, demanding
    bulge in my body
    that I have grown to love so well,

I pray God will safely guide you
    on your journey tonight
    and I ask Him for the strength
    to help you all I can.

Again you signal
    your impatience
    to be set free.
    Time to wake your Daddy.

TO YOU, MY CHILD

A Parent's Reflection

If there could be only one thing in life for me to teach you, I would teach you to

LOVE...

To respect others so that you may find respect in yourself. To learn the value of giving, so that if ever there comes a time in your life that someone really needs,

YOU WILL GIVE.

To act in a manner that you would wish to be treated: to be proud of yourself. To LAUGH and SMILE, as much as you can, in order to help bring joy back into this world. To have FAITH in others.

To stand tall in this world and to learn to depend on yourself. To only take from this earth those things which you really need. To not depend on money or material things for your happiness, but to learn to appreciate people who love you, the simple beauty that GOD gave you and to find peace and security within yourself.

TO YOU, MY CHILD, I hope I have taught all these things, for they are LOVE.

AUTHOR'S NOTES

Special Deliveries, the author, publisher, any doctors, nurses, religious, or any affiliated hospitals and/or products are not responsible for the outcome of actions taken according to the information contained in this book. This information is solely a diagrammatical record of experience and knowledge the author acquired during her own extensive research on the subject of gender selection. The method has worked for the author three times in a row, and also for others, all over the world, which is proving the method's effectiveness.

Please feel free to send along your own individual success stories, which this book may have helped make possible, along with the data to show evidence of following this method. Refer to *Special Deliveries* Scientifically Controlled Study on page 101 of this book.

S⦿URCES

1. SETTLES, LANDRUM B., MD, PHD
   & DAVID M. RORVIK

   "How to Choose the Sex of Your Baby"

2. CURTIS, LINDSAY R., MD
   & YVONNE COROLES, RN

   "Pregnant and Loving It..."

3. NEWSWEEK
   FEBRUARY, 1975

   "Coital Patterns Successful in Predicting Child's Sex"

4. TIME
   JUNE, 1960

   "Toward Sex in Order"

5. SCIENCE DIGEST
   APRIL, 1974

   "Boy or Girl, Take Your Pick"

6. UNDERSTANDING PREGNANCY AND CHILDBIRTH

   Sheldon H. Cherry, M.D., 1992

7. TAKING CHARGE OF YOUR FERTILITY

   Toni Weschler, 1995

TESTIMONIALS

I continue to hear from people all over the world on a regular basis, both by phone, fax and mail, attesting that the *"Special Deliveries"* method has worked for them. I once heard from a woman in Naples, Florida who had purchased the book back in 1992. She had one daughter at the time, who just turned four years old. Because of some medical complications, she was deterred from trying for a son she and her husband longed for (her husband is William the 4th). Once her doctor gave her the approval to start trying for a baby, she followed my method.

She called me very excited about her doctor's visit for her five month check-up. She had a routine ultrasound done which confirmed she was carrying their son, William the 5th (pictured on page 87).

It is stories like these and countless others that make me realize that we are all on this earth to help and learn from each other. I believe I am helping alleviate some of the disappointments that many people have expressed when they have 2, 3 or more children of the same gender. The following testimonials are just a few of the countless letters I have received that continue to attest to the success rate of this method.

The following are a compilation of just a few of the countless testimonials *"Special Deliveries"* continues to receive.

My husband and I always planned on having three children. After our two sons were born, we knew that we wanted only one more child and if we could have a girl, we'd be thrilled. We followed *"Special Deliveries"* instructions, which were easy, safe and natural.

When I ultimately delivered my daughter, Maris, born February 1995, I kept asking the doctor in the delivery room if it was really a girl. I believe this method really works and would highly recommend it to anyone.

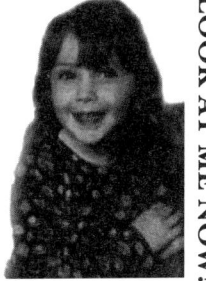

LOOK AT ME NOW!

MARLENE OLIVIER
Bellmore, New York

ॐॐ

Our first child was a very special, beautiful girl. Due to our busy lifestyles we wanted only two children, so of course, we hoped for a boy as our second child. To increase our odds we purchased *"Special Deliveries"*. We read it, followed the easy-to-follow methods and on May 11, 1994 we delivered a healthy baby boy, our son, Brandon Bolach.

LOOK AT ME NOW!

We truly believe *"Special Deliveries"* methods help you choose the sex of your child! Thank you for your publication. Thanks to *"Special Deliveries"*, we have our desired family.

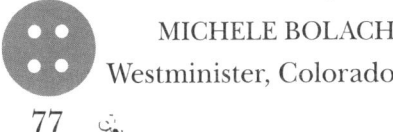

MICHELE BOLACH
Westminister, Colorado

We are all very happy and would like to thank you so much for your information. We had three boys and thanks to *"Special Deliveries"* our family is now complete with our daughter to add "sugar & spice & everything nice" to our lives.

PATRICIA & ROBERT BAKER
Greenville, Pennsylvania

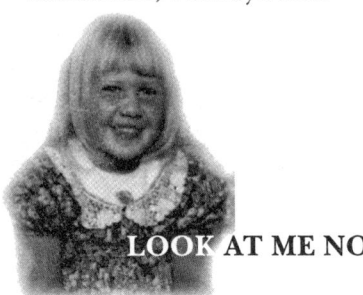

LOOK AT ME NOW!

⤙⤚

My husband comes from a family of four brothers who had a total of twelve (12) daughters and only one (1) son between them. My in-laws were about to give up on having any more grandsons when I ordered your book. The family was all pretty skeptical until our son, Colton Toren, was born in February of 1994.

Now my sister-in-law wants to try for a boy using your methods: they have three girls.

I have told everyone I know about *"Special Deliveries"*. I am a true believer!! Keep up the good work.

LAURA TOREN
Sun River, Montana

Thank you for making the information available. Without your book, the odds were against us to conceive a girl. My husband is one of seven brothers and only one sister. Boys dominate in the Bedwell family. Our daughter Anna Chantelle Bedwell was born in April of 1994. Also, a friend had borrowed my book and used it before me. She tried for a boy and the result was a boy. He was born in February of 1994. Their family is now complete as they have two daughters and their " *Special Deliveries*" son.

ABBIE BEDWELL
Lawrenceville, Illinois

೮∾ಳಿ LOOK AT ME NOW!

My husband and I greatly enjoyed your book, "*Special Deliveries*". The methods described in your book have already worked for us twice and we plan to use it again. Having a brother to grow up with, my husband always wanted two sons. I am from a family of two girls and I know, no matter how many friends you have, there is nothing like having a sister. There were five (5) girls born on my husband's side and my boys were the most welcome grandsons.

I do think this is a sound method and believe in it instead of high tech, morally questionable gender selection procedures. Your book provides an excellent and ethical choice to gender selection. We enjoyed trying for our two sons and will try again soon for two girls. *(As seen on the nationally syndicated Mike & Maty show, televised February, 1996.)*

DR. & MRS. J. MASSARSKY
Centerville, Massachusetts

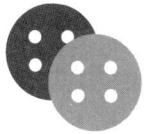

My first pregnancy resulted in the birth of our son, Drew, born in September. Three months later, I was pregnant again and our second son, Cole, was born the following September. We were tempted to stop at two healthy boys, but decided to try once more, hoping for a baby girl this time. This was when we first heard about *"Special Deliveries"*. *"Special Deliveries"* made sense to us and we wanted to increase our odds, if at all possible.

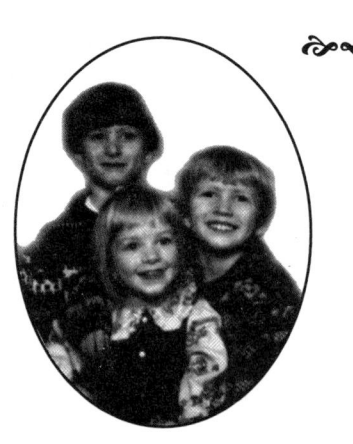

After months of timing, it finally happened. That September, when Cole was two and Drew would be three, Emma was born. What a delightful surprise!. It had worked for us. We now have three beautiful children, two boys and one girl.

ELAINE LEDWITH
East Swanzey, New Hampshire

ॐॐ

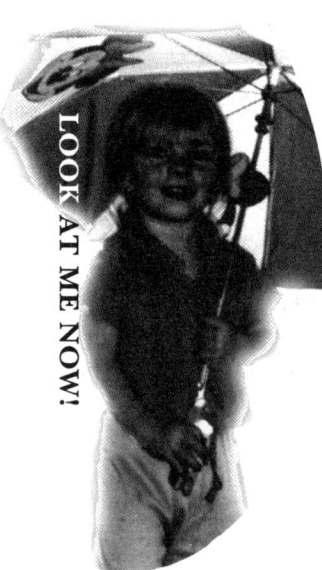

LOOK AT ME NOW!

Seven years ago I had a beautiful baby girl, but I knew that I would like to have another baby and that my husband would love to have a son. In 1990, I had a serious back injury and thought that I would not be able to have another baby. Fortunately, I started feeling stronger with physical therapy, etc. and decided that it was my last chance to try for a son.

I certainly had no time or energy after all my back trouble to go to the local library or bookstores to do research myself never mind decipher which would work. Then I remembered a book entitled *"Special Deliveries"* that a friend had given me after she used it successfully. After reading it and reviewing it, to work we went.

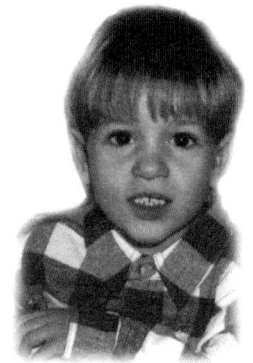

Happily on November 16th, 1994 at 5:36 a.m., we were holding our beautiful, healthy, very Special Delivery son, Felipe. My friend, myself, our husbands and families agree that it was well worth the cost of your book, for a lifetime of enjoyment with our babies! Thank you for enhancing our chances to conceive the baby of our choice.

CONNIE JONET-BRANCO
Brockton, Massachusetts

LOOK AT ME NOW!

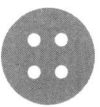

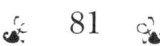

I very happily saw the author Theresa Hebert on national television. I am delighted with my 2 year old son, Keoni and I knew in my heart I longed to share my life with a daughter as well. What Theresa said on television made so much sense. So I immediately purchased *"Special Deliveries"* and I got the opportunity to speak with Theresa herself. I was very anxious and she very nicely calmed all my fears and explained her theory. She said with the knowledge and some patience it could work for me as it had for so many others. I am so thankful I listened to her suggestions. You need to apply yourself and take your time, because all good things come to those who wait. Thank you again. We are enjoying our beautiful little girl so much. Our family is originally from Hawaii so we named our daughter, Kamalani, which in Hawaiian means "the child from Heaven." We truly feel blessed and believe Theresa is an angel for helping so many others just like us. We will always be grateful for her sharing of this information with others.

Ilia Kaku
Los Angeles, California

Thank you so much, *"Special Deliveries"*, for the information you provided in your book. I truly believe in the theory behind conceiving a boy or girl and the easy to follow instructions made conceiving fun, not pressure!

My husband and I wanted a little brother for our daughter Alexis and thanks to *"Special Deliveries"*, our little Andrew was born 4 days ago, August 1997.

Thanks again!

John & Kristen
Ciacciarelli

Cranston, Rhode Island

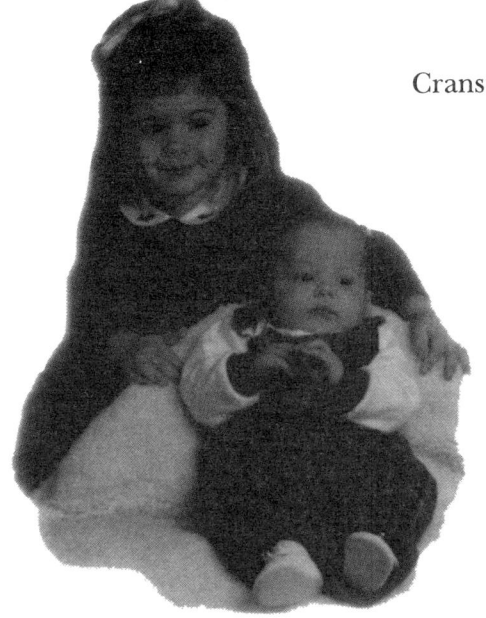

As seen on CNN television and heard on 92 Pro-FM radio, Providence R.I. Oct.1997

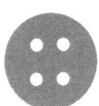

When my husband and I decided to have a second child we thought, "Wouldn't it be nice to have a girl this time?". Out of twelve grandchildren on both sides, there were only two girls. We thought our chances were pretty slim. Ironically, on our son, Kevin's, second birthday I saw Theresa Hebert on television promoting her book. I immediately went out, bought the book, read it (re-read it) and even talked to Theresa on the phone for advice and guidance. On January 19, 1997 our beautiful daughter Megan Claire Kathryn was born! I was so completely sold on her theory that I told my sister, who is now expecting and have told all my friends. I am a true believer! Thank you, Theresa, for making our dreams possible!

Fondly,

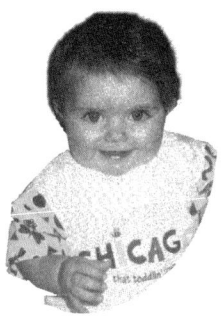

Steve & Karen Peyton
Breckenridge, Colorado

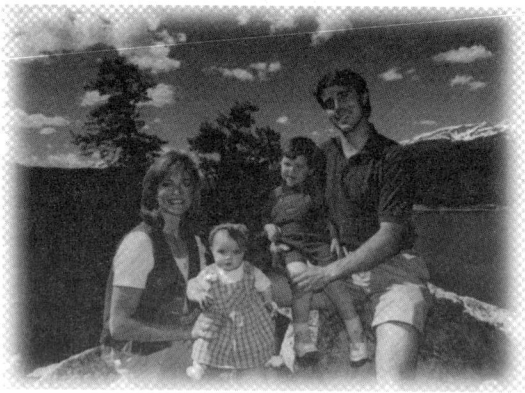

No one can express the excitement and joy my husband and I felt when we had our little boy, Connor Patrick MacJack, 8 1/4 lbs. on October 1st, 1997. We have a lovely 2 year old daughter Brenna Kathleen and we really wanted a boy. We followed the instructions and had our little boy! We plan to use the book next time.

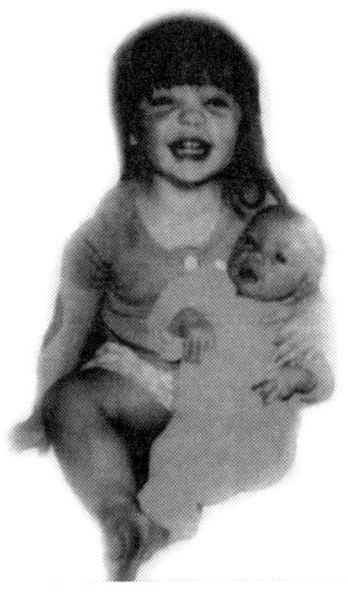

Tracy MacJack
Woodstock, Georgia

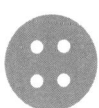

I am looking at my 2 month old baby daughter as I write this letter. If it were not for your book I believe she would not be here today. We have two healthy sons named Matthew, 4 1/2 and Nathan, 2 1/2. We thought we only wanted to have two children, but then when Nathan was born, my desire for a daughter slowly grew. We discussed having a third child and felt it was financially possible and a daughter would complete our family.

I heard about your book on national television back in February 1996. I finally got your address and information in the mail and I sent for your book March 9, 1996. We anxiously awaited the book and fervently read it through many times. I took my temperature and kept the charts for several months. My husband Glenn was very patient and understanding. In April, we conceived and nine months later Rachel was born. When I was 24 weeks pregnant I had an ultrasound the technician said she was 98% sure I was having a girl. I was never sure until the doctor delivered Rachel and told me, "It's a girl!". Those were beautiful words to hear and now Rachel Elizabeth Lawson completes our family of five along with her two big brothers, Matthew and Nathan.

Thank you so much for your book. Please make it more available to the public. Also, many of the women I work with are interested in the method. Thank you again for your research and information.

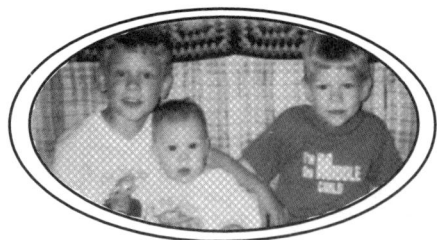

Michelle Lawson
Chicago, Illinois

& via&

My daughter Kayla Marie was born in 1990. We were delighted with our new bundle of joy and as our time with her enlightened our lives, we realized we wanted one more child - a boy to carry on the William Tyler Douglass tradition. In a magazine I saw an article for your book and I purchased it. For one year I charted my temperature and compared each month, not really trying to conceive. Unfortunately, we had no success and thought we should go to a specialist to determine the reason for not conceiving.

Shortly after, I was diagnosed with endometriosis and had a laproscopy done. My physician indicated that things were all clear and that it should not take very long for conception to occur, but not to be discouraged if it did not.

On October 13, 1995 I began my menstrual cycle. It was a four day cycle. I then patiently began to chart my temperature. My husband and I decided to try your method for three months, then revert back to "Hey, it's ovulation time...come on!" On the 14th day of my cycle I ovulated and had intercourse only on that day, since my husband was out of town.

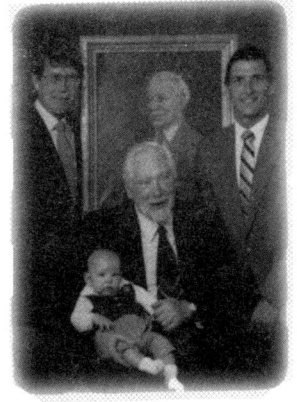

How excited I was when the tube of the pregnancy test turned color. I was pregnant. "Hooray!"

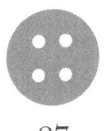

In March I had an ultrasound and the doctor identified our son very clearly on the sonagram. Last week the doctor indicated by the ultrasound that we should indeed have a son in July of this year. I have recommended your book and method to many people. I truly believe if someone follows your book practices and really wants to try to assist nature in their selection of the sex of their child it can be accomplished.

5th generation
William Tyler Douglass V
Born: July 26, 1996

Sincerely,
Lisa Douglass
Naples, Florida

I am presently the mother of two boys, ages 6 and 2. My husband and I were happy with the size of our family, but were encouraged to try for the little girl we always wanted after I saw your appearance on the "Mike and Maty" show last spring. I began charting my ovulation as your book suggests when I saw a segment on "Dateline" which refuted the methods of gender selection that you were proposing. The segment went on to feature a doctor who was doing work in the area of sperm separation and who was having certain successes in gender selection. My husband and I went to see this doctor who told us that with his method, my chances of conceiving a girl would go from 49% naturally to 75%. He also said that I would need to start taking the fertility drug Clomid and that my chances of conceiving twins would almost double! As I am already in an age group with a higher chance of multiple births (over 35) which we did not want, and also because I am a migraine headache sufferer and was afraid of side effects, I did not want to start taking the Clomid and we opted out of the procedure.

So I went back to the natural method proposed in your book and in September became pregnant. My amniocentesis performed this past December confirmed that we were having our little girl in early June. Thank you Theresa for staying out there, publicizing your research in the face of skeptics who simply cannot refute the success stories you have been documenting over the years.

Wishing you and your family health and happiness.

Jenna Layne
Born on June 5, 1997

Kim R.
Merrick, New York

In July of 1996 I heard the author on **92-Pro-FM** radio with Mike Butts in the morning. I was so interested in listening to what she was saying because my husband and I had been talking about starting a family soon and we both hoped to start our family with a son. I come from a family with just two girls and never had a brother and we had no grandsons on my parents' side of the family, so they hoped for a grandson as well. I purchased the book right away at a local book store, read the book and followed the method. At 20 weeks along, I had a routine ultrasound and was ecstatically happy to find out that indeed I was carrying our son and on November 23, 1997 our first born Tyler Edward was born weighing in at 8 lbs. 13 oz. I think it's wonderful that Theresa took the time to write a book that makes it possible for couples everywhere to have an active role in actually planning their families. Thank you for sharing this information and giving people everywhere a natural alternative to family planning.

KIM PIETRZYK
Raynham, Massachusetts

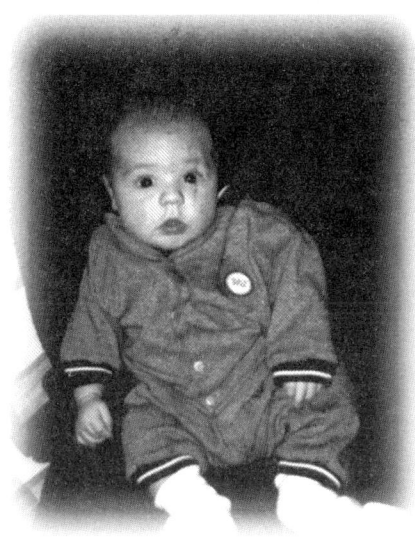

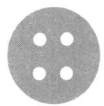

In 1993 my husband Brian and I were married. I was 32 years old at the time and because of my age and a family history of medical complications was anxious to start a family right away. One year prior to our wedding we met the author of *"Special Deliveries"*, Theresa Hebert, at a Christmas party. I spoke with Theresa and told her of our plans to start a family very soon after we married and how we both hoped for a son. She shared the first edition of her book with us and I must say at the time I was somewhat skeptical. However, soon after reading the book my husband and I agreed that the method she described made sense in many ways, including scientifically. We decided to try for the little boy of our dreams. When our son Jacob was born on July 8, 1994 we were so very happy. In 1996 we began discussing the possibility of having one more child and using the *"Special Deliveries"* book once again. Again we followed the instructions, but this time for a baby girl; and lo and behold our beautiful daughter Victoria was born on May 6, 1997. Needless to say I am no longer skeptical and let friends and family know about this very "Special" book. As I said on national television on "Inside Edition" in October 1997, I am now 100% convinced in the *"Special Deliveries"* method and feel it is important to let others know they also have the same opportunity to increase their chances of planning their future families if they so desire.

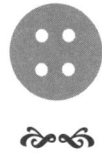

JOAN GOMES
Massachusetts

(As seen on national television's INSIDE EDITION *October 1997*)

❧❧

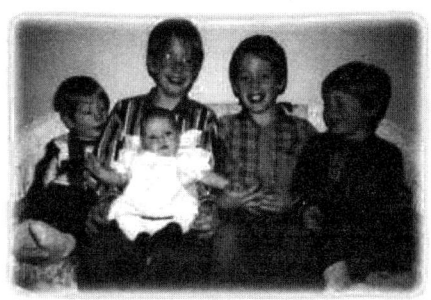

My husband and I were blessed with four wonderful sons. However, I have always pictured us with a daughter in our family. I ordered the *"Special Deliveries"* book and after reading, studying and following the method once, we were both confident and understood what to do. We decided then that we were ready to actually start trying and very happily became pregnant. This pregnancy was 100% different from the last four in many ways. Then at 20 weeks, my ultrasound said I was carrying a girl, our daughter. Our dream came true on August 21, 1997 when our little princess, "Jillian Barbara Hecker" was born 7 lbs. 7 ozs. Our boys love their little sister so much! Thanks to God and the availability of Theresa's book, we now have a "Special Deliveries" baby girl to complete our family. We are not ready to put *"Special Deliveries"* book away just yet. This may sound funny, but sometimes I think it would be nice for Jillian to someday have a sister.

As featured in the Chicago News Sun Paper

Chicago, Illinois (December 10, 1997)

కొడంశ్

Mari Jo Hecker

Elmhurst, Illinois

We are so very happy and proud of our little boy Derek, born on February 10, 1998. Our girls absolutely love him. Ariana, our 3 year old, is a little mother to him. Ariel is still a little too young to pay as much attention just yet.

After reading your book over and over again to make sure that I understood everything and charting for several months and even consulting with you by phone, we conceived our son. (Thank you, by the way, for telling me to take my time and be patient; he certainly was well worth the wait.)

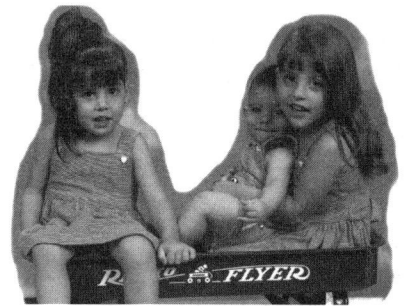

If you could only have seen my husband's face when the doctor said, "It's a boy!" He couldn't believe it, neither could I. We were elated!!

Theresa, thank you for writing such a helpful, informative book and yet simple enough for anyone to understand and follow.

I'm very happy that I had the opportunity to read your book and have more information about choosing the gender of our baby before conception especially since we both honestly wanted a baby boy so badly after being lucky enough to have two beautiful little girls.

George, Lucy
Ariana, Ariel and
"Special Delivery" Derek Pereira
Massachusetts

(As seen on nationally syndicated television's **"Smart Woman"**, Ivanhoe Broadcast News, Inc. September 1998.)

My husband and I always hoped to have two children. We were blessed with a son Danny, our firstborn, and realized someday in the future we would love to have another. We honestly thought how wonderful it would be to have a daughter, since we would probably only plan on having two children.

Before considering trying for our second child, I turned to my sister Karen Peyton, (pictured on page 84 with her family) because she had followed the expert advice of Theresa Hebert and her book "**Special Deliveries**" to successfully conceive her daughter. I not only read the book, but also consulted with Theresa personally.

The method was very easy to follow, not to mention safe and inexpensive. I also had the extra confidence of knowing the book had already worked for my sister and some of her friends as well.

With the guidance of Theresa and her book and a blessing from God, we had our second child on July 4, 1998, our daughter Claire Marie, at 4:50 p.m. weighing in at 7 lbs., 20 in.! I am so thrilled to have two special and healthy children. What a joy to have the experience of sharing our lives with a son as well as a daughter.

Thank you, Theresa, for giving people everywhere the knowledge of other options, so they can make their own decision based on what is best for them. We can now all testify, (my sister, myself, and friends) that the "Special Deliveries" method really does work, because we (all educated women who really knew our bodies) now all have living proof!!!

Jane and Mike Cvengros
LaGrange, IL

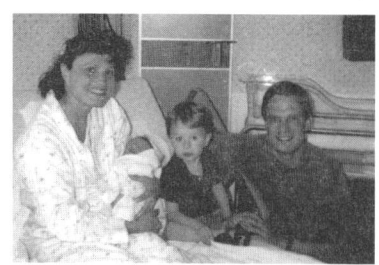

☙ 93 ❧

In December of 1993 we had our first child, our son John Peter; we were extremely elated. We knew having another child would make our family complete, especially if that child were a girl.

In November of 1996, after previously seeing the author, Theresa Hebert on national television, I phoned her office to find out where I would be able to purchase her book, "<u>Special Deliveries</u>."

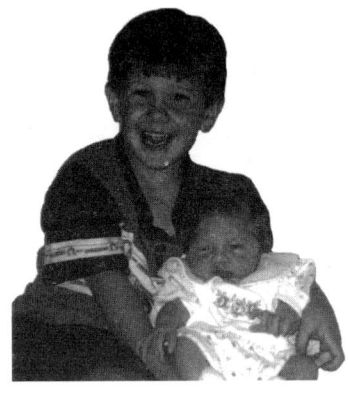

After many telephone consultations, patience, and perseverance, I conceived our second child in September of 1997. Our beautiful "Special Delivery" daughter Nicole Grace, was born on June 14, 1998. Nicole Grace has surely brightened our lives, especially for her big brother John Peter.

We thank you, Theresa, for your time, care, sincerity, love and support. Nicole is truly our "Special Deliveries" baby. Our family is now complete. Thank you again for everything.

The Grzymalskis
Lenore, Peter
John Peter
and "Special Delivery" Nicole Grace
New Hyde Park, New York

(As seen on national television's **ABC's "The View" with Barbara Walters** September 11, 1998.)

Before, During and After Pregnancy...

BETTER HEALTH THROUGH RELIV®

♦ Receive optimal nutrition

♦ Lose weight safely

♦ Boost immune system and energy levels

♦ Achieve maximum physical performance

♦ Enhance mental productivity

♦ Maintain a healthy weight

♦ Work at home around your family's schedule

"With Reliv you can reach your peak performance level and achieve permanent weight loss. I have received the benefits of the Reliv program for more than four years now, and I highly recommend it to anyone wanting to feel happy, healthy, and energetic. What parent doesn't want that?"

> Theresa Hebert
> Author, Special Deliveries

For information about Reliv® products or the Reliv® business opportunity call:
Mary Monteiro
Independent Reliv® Distributor #097-359
1-800-517-9280
(Mention Code SD 98-3)
Or simply mail the coupon below.

- -

Information Request

Name _____

Address_____

_____Zip_____

Tel: (Home)_____ (Work)_____

🖌 Please check all areas of interest:

___ A natural approach to a health problem	___ More energy
___ Safe, easy weight loss	___ Nutrition as prevention
___ Nutritional support during pregnancy	___ Introduce a friend to Reliv®
___ Part-time supplemental income	___ Full-time career helping others

Mail to:
Mary Monteiro
Independent Reliv® Distributor ID#097-359
29 Medeiros Lane
North Dartmouth, MA 02747
Tel: 1-800-517-9280

The Two Most Frequently Asked Questions of The Author; When Trying To Conceive A Child.

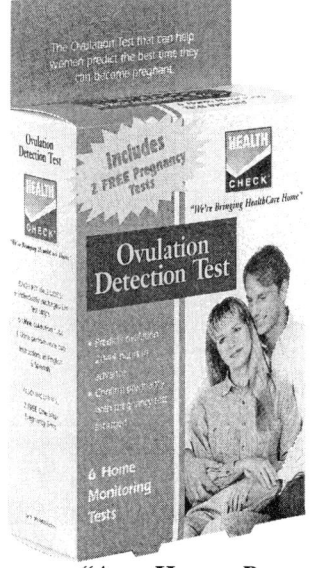

"Which Home Ovulation Detection Test do you recommend?"

I am very happy to introduce the HealthCheck™ Home Ovulation Detection Kit. This product offers a high quality, very affordable at-home test for predicting ovulation 20-44 hours in advance. The kit contains six ovulation tests and as a bonus two free pregnancy tests! The HealthCheck™ Ovulation Kit contains enough strips for 6 days of testing, increasing the chance of detecting an LH surge by 10% vs. similar products on the market.

"Are Home Pregnancy tests really as accurate as the pregnancy test done in a laboratory or doctor's office?"

YES!!! Over the past ten years there have been tremendous strides in pregnancy test technology. This has led to greatly improved quality and reliability in these tests. Today's tests are 99% accurate, and can detect pregnancy as early as one day after a missed period. I recommend the HealthCheck™ One-Step One Minute Pregnancy Test.

You get accurate results in just 60 seconds. Early detection of pregnancy is essential to allow for early prenatal care, and this test is so sensitive it can detect pregnancy as early as 1 day after your missed period unlike other national brands.

Today's consumers are looking for ways to exert more control over their lives and their health and home diagnostic tests enable them to do so. These products are <u>accurate,</u> <u>quick,</u> and <u>inexpensive</u>. **For more information** on any of the HealthCheck™ products including the Home Ovulation Detection Test and how to purchase a kit yourself, simply contact Special Deliveries at **(508) 880-7848**.

Do you have friends or relatives who would like to have copies of this book? If so, please fill in the order blank below or call to order.

ORDER FORM

Please send_____ copies of

"Special Deliveries" at $19.95 each to:

(Add $4.99 Shipping & Handling)

Name:_____

Address:_____

City:_____

State:_____Zip:_____

Telephone: (____)_____

MAKE CHECK OR MONEY ORDER PAYABLE TO:

SPECIAL DELIVERIES

67 SOUTH CRANE AVENUE
DEPT. BK98-3
TAUNTON, MA 02780
(508) 880-7848
or CALL TOLL FREE: (888) 688-7728
TO ORDER WITH A MAJOR CREDIT CARD

Do you have friends or relatives who would like to have copies of this book? If so, please fill in the order blank below or call to order.

ORDER FORM

Please send_____ copies of

"Special Deliveries" at $19.95 each to:

(Add $4.99 Shipping & Handling)

Name:_____

Address:_____

City:_____

State:_____Zip:_____

Telephone: (____)_____

MAKE CHECK OR MONEY ORDER PAYABLE TO:
SPECIAL DELIVERIES

67 SOUTH CRANE AVENUE
DEPT. BK98-3
TAUNTON, MA 02780
(508) 880-7848
or CALL TOLL FREE: (888) 688-7728
TO ORDER WITH A MAJOR CREDIT CARD

HOW TO BE INCLUDED IN THE SCIENTIFICALLY CONTROLLED STUDY

If you would like to be included in *"Special Deliveries"* scientifically controlled studies, simply send along a copy of your own individual BBT charting and / or your Ovulation Predictor Test Charting, both specifically from the month you actually conceived your baby. Include your name, address, telephone, signature, dates, etc. and send them along with the **"Special Deliveries"** Survey Update (filled out by you), from this book. It is that simple. This information is considered DATA for any doctors or affiliated hospitals to view and come to their conclusions in regards to this method. Thank you.

Please feel free to send *"Special Deliveries"* your success stories, which this book may have helped make possible. Baby pictures are always welcome.

SPECIAL DELIVERIES SURVEY

Name:_____

Address:_____

City:_____

State:_____Zip:_____

Telephone (____)_____

Approximately, when did you purchase this book?_____

_____

Did you read and follow the methods as directed?_____

_____

Did the results work in your favor?_____

How many children did you have before using *"Special Deliveries"*? (please list name(s), age(s), gender)

_____
_____
_____

After reading **"Special Deliveries"**, did you conceive? (please list name(s), age(s), gender)

_____
_____
_____

Do you or your family have any comments or suggestions for *"Special Deliveries?"*

Please mail survey to: *"Special Deliveries"* **Attn: Survey Dept. 98-3**
67 South Crane Ave., Taunton, MA 02780

Or simply FAX or call your results in at (508)880-7848

WE'D LOVE TO HEAR FROM YOU!

FIGURE 1: BASAL BODY TEMPERATURE INSTRUCTIONS

FIGURE 1: BASAL BODY TEMPERATURE INSTRUCTIONS

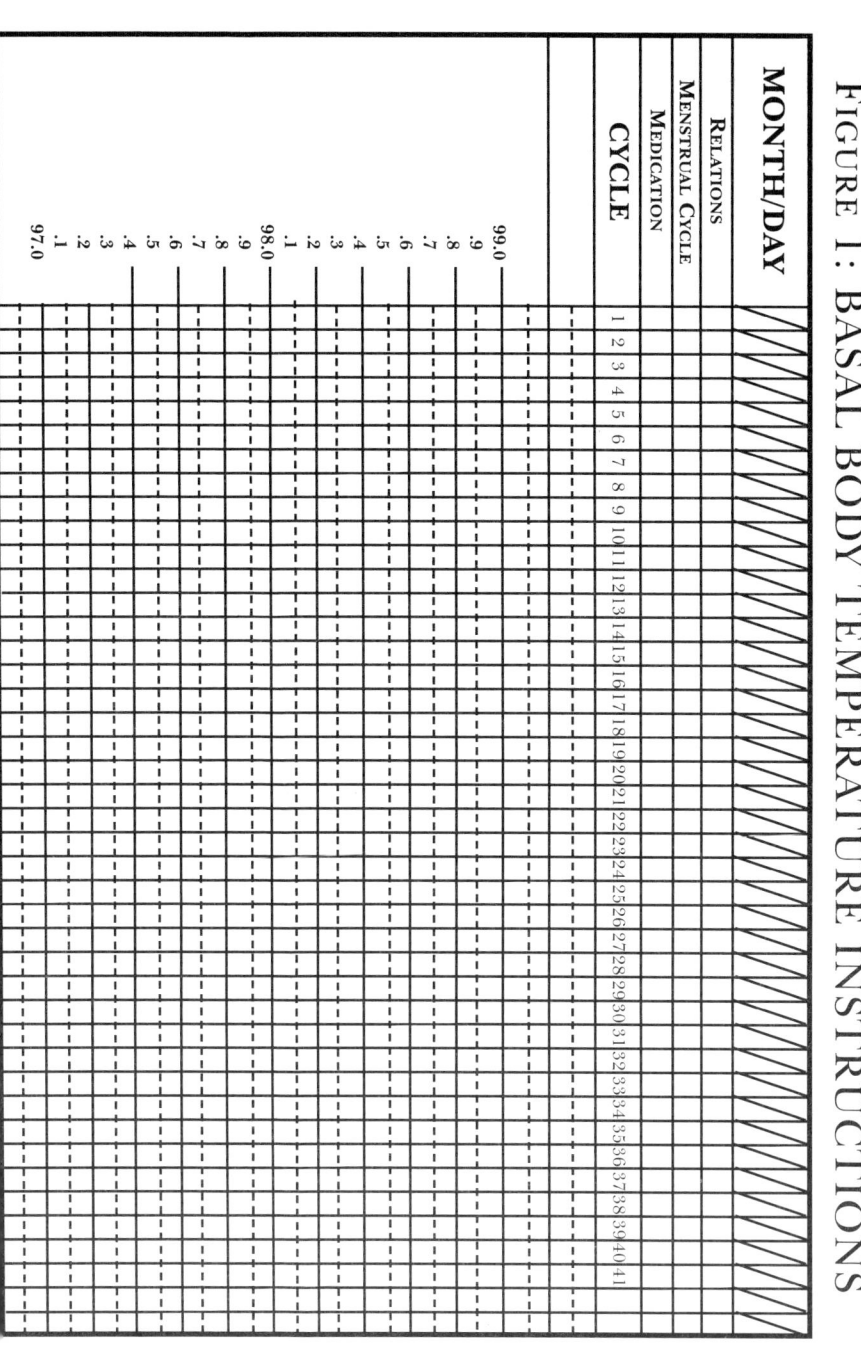

SUMMARY

Did you know there are actual ways to improve your chances of conceiving the child of your preference?

Whether this is your first baby, or your fourth, chances are you've heard some of these remarks before:

"Are you hoping for a boy or a girl?"

"I bet you want a boy this time!"

"Are you trying for a girl?"

In the early 1980's a doctor told me because of ovarian fibroid cysts and a tipped uterus, I might have trouble conceiving a child. I immediately started reading, studying and questioning for the answers to conceive and while researching, stumbled upon the subject of gender selection. I then put together a **safe, easy and completely natural method** that I followed and conceived the child of my preference, not once, but **three times** and delivered all three children on their due dates. This method has nothing to do with diet, positioning or the use of unnatural substances. **Again, it is safe, easy and natural!**

Having kept extensive records for each of my three pregnancies, I was convinced that these methods worked for me and would, in turn, work for others as well. I wrote the book in 1990 right after my daughter was born to share with others this information. This book has been actively sold since 1990 and in January of 1995, I started corresponding with couples who used the book. Overwhelming results showed that the people who read the book and followed its method, also conceived the child of their preference. The copyright was received on March 30, 1995.

I've since received letters from people all over the world, including California, New York, Texas, Canada, Hawaii, Puerto Rico, even Saudi Arabia and Lebanon all with a **NATURAL HUMAN DESIRE** for one gender over the other. These feelings are universal.

Laura Toren, of **Sun River, Montana**, was thrilled to deliver her son Colten in February of 1994 after having had three daughters. Her husband's side of the family had 12 granddaughters. So, they were thrilled with a boy to carry on their name.

Patricia and Robert Baker of **Greenville, Pennsylvania**, had three boys, read *"Special Deliveries"* and now have a healthy baby girl to complete their family.

Valerie and Craig Underhill of **McLean, Virginia**, said, *"When we purchased 'Special Deliveries' book we had only one son at the time. Due to our busy working careers that included travel, we planned on only having two children and really wanted a girl for our second child. We believe based on statistics and the methodology devised by Theresa Hebert that the reason we have our daughter today, is due to her publication. We would like to thank her for making this book available!"*

The list of testimonials goes on and on. My reason for writing this book was simple. There seems to be a universal experience among couples bearing their first child. People automatically assume they'll want the opposite gender the second time around. Comments abound to that effect, and of course, it gets worse when they have two, three or more of the same gender. In today's fast-paced society, where in some cases both parents work outside as well as inside the home, they would rather not leave to chance the desired gender of their baby.

COMMENTS FROM THE MEDICAL COMMUNITY

Doctors' opinions have varied yet some doctors are now willing to offer *"Special Deliveries"* as an option to their patients and let them formulate their own ideas and make their own educated decisions as to what is best for them.

As one medical expert said to me on the phone, *"I would very much like to be included in the process of helping educate the couples of today and be an important part of teaching them this invaluable information that I believe is on the verge of making medical history."*

One OB-GYN doctor from Massachusetts stated in a recent newspaper article, ***"Special Deliveries"*** method offers several advantages. It is safe, non-invasive, inexpensive and easy to follow. While nothing is 100% guaranteed, there are patients who express an interest in influencing their baby's gender.

"We refer patients to the *"Special Deliveries"* book as an alternative if they have already decided they want to add to their family and would welcome any baby into their home."

"We are very interested in further studying this safe, non-invasive technique for sex selection. I feel it is a great alternative for couples to plan their families!"

While another doctor stated, "I feel it's important to be open to alternative methods."

Another doctor from California on television with the author stated, "There is absolutely no harm or risk to this method."

It is so thrilling to be able to share this very much desired information with people who would lovingly welcome any baby into their homes, but planning to have another child anyway, are now able to enhance their chances by taking it one simple, easy step further. **Doctor Jack Massarsky and wife Lorraine of Centerville, Massachusetts**, said, *"Your book was a wonderful alternative and most ethical solution to our planned family of two boys and someday in the future two girls."* **This couple also appeared on the Mike and Maty Show on February 13, 1996.**

"We were so happy when we heard you on 92 Pro-FM radio in July of 1996. We had always hoped for a son after having had our beautiful daughter. We now know we are not alone when we express our feelings about what 'Special Deliveries' helped us accomplish. It is so wonderful to be able to experience not only what it's like to have a daughter, but a son as well. We were very grateful and happy to share our success story on television, as well as radio in October of 1997." **Kristen and John Ciacciarelli appeared on CNN television with their family, daughter Alexis and their "Special Delivery" son, Andrew, born in August of 1997.**

One of the many things I have learned in the 15 years of research is that one couple's idea of the perfect family can be quite different from another. But they have all agreed that because of the availability of information in this book, which was easy to follow and got right to the point, they conceived their desired families.

On December 20, 1997 I received a thank you card from a woman in Oregon who just had an ultrasound done, which confirmed she will be having her much dreamed of little girl, due March 12, 1998 after 4 boys.

Her story and others like hers is precisely why I continue to share this information with interested people around the globe. To know that simply by sharing knowledge that I have acquired can actually help make them aware that indeed they can play an active role in planning their families, is unequivocally one of the most gratifying feelings in the world for me.

I first consulted with this woman back in November of 1996 when she first expressed to me her strong desire for a daughter. She was a pleasure to speak with and a woman of strong spiritual faith who was one of the first to express her feeling that God helps those who help themselves. She said, "if His plan was for her to someday have a daughter, she surely would."

" Anything that enlarges the sphere of human powers that shows man he can do what he thought he could not do, is valuable, and that makes 'Special Deliveries' very valuable."

"YOU DON'T NEED MY HELP ANY LONGER, YOU'VE ALWAYS HAD THE POWER."

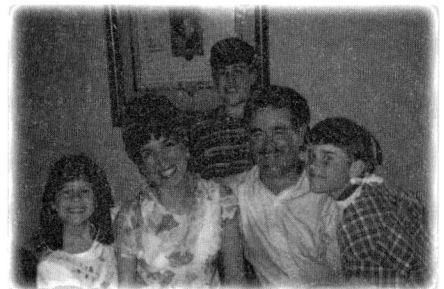

Theresa with her family at her grandmother's 90th Birthday Celebration.

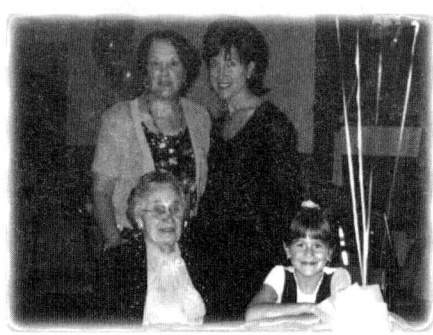

Four generations of women at Theresa's recent 40th birthday celebration.

◆ *Bella Vaz*
◆ *Elsie Vaz Ducharme*
◆ *Theresa Vaz Ducharme Hebert*
◆ *"Special Delivery"* Baby:
    Arielle Elena
    Vaz Ducharme Hebert

Theresa while in New York City taping, "Lifetime Television for Women"

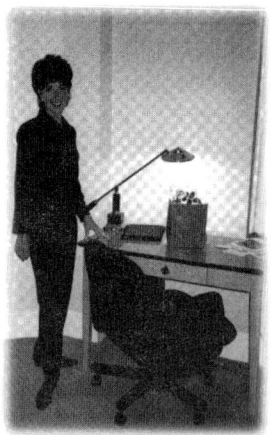